The Evaluation and Care of

SEVERELY DISTURBED CHILDREN

and Their Families

The Evaluation and Care of

SEVERELY DISTURBED CHILDREN

and Their Families

Edited By
LEON HOFFMAN, M.D.
Psychiatrist-In-Charge
Inpatient Unit
Assistant Clinical Professor
Mount Sinai School of Medicine
New York, New York

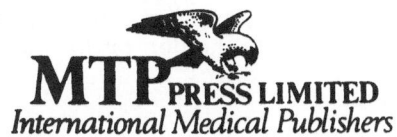
MTP **PRESS LIMITED**
International Medical Publishers

Published in the UK and Europe by
MTP Press Limited
Falcon House
Lancaster, England

Published in the US by
SPECTRUM PUBLICATIONS, INC.
175-20 Wexford Terrace
Jamaica, N.Y. 11432

ISBN-13: 978-94-011-6301-9   e-ISBN-13: 978-94-011-6299-9
DOI: 10.1007/ 978-94-011-6299-9

ACKNOWLEDGEMENT

I would like to acknowledge the hard work of all the contributors to this volume. I am most grateful to Mortimer Blumenthal, M.D., Acting Director of Child and Adolescent Psychiatry at the Mount Sinai Medical Center for his encouragement and careful reading of the manuscript. Dr. Irving Berlin, Director, Division of Child and Adolescent Psychiatry at the University of New Mexico Medical School, Albuquerque, New Mexico, was very kind in critically reading the manuscript and suggesting various changes. I would like to thank Marvin Stein, M.D., Professor and Chairman, Department of Psychiatry at the Mount Sinai Medical Center for his support. The secretarial staff of the Department of Psychiatry was helpful and efficient. I would like to especially thank Ms. Mary Carter and Ms. Louise Chapman.

Finally, and most importantly, a special note of appreciation must be given to the permanent staff of "6 South" and the Day Treatment Program. To them this volume is dedicated. Their untiring devotion to the children is a gift to be treasured.

Leon Hoffman, M.D.

ACKNOWLEDGEMENT

FOREWORD

This book, which proposes a developmental view of short-term inpatient treatment for severely disturbed children, is much needed in our field. It is particularly relevant, emotionally engaging, and a pleasure to read because the writers who are the actual participants and leaders in the milieu program, discuss their own experiences with a variety of children. The principles of milieu therapy are beautifully described and its application to a diverse ethnic population of sick children is clearly delineated.

I congratulate Leon Hoffman and his co-workers for bringing to the field of child psychiatry a timely and helpful work.

Irving N. Berlin, M.D.
Professor of Psychiatry and Pediatrics
Director, Division of Child and
Adolescent Psychiatry, and Director,
Children's Psychiatric Center,
University of New Mexico School of
Medicine, Albuquerque, New Mexico

PREFACE

Children who require hospital or residential treatment need an
environment that provides a structure to their daily activities. Much
of the literature on milieu treatment is inadequate because of a lack of
integration between the various theoretical frames of reference and their
practical application. Berlin has stressed the importance of a developmental frame of reference in the organization of a hospital child
psychiatry unit.*

The Mount Sinai Medical Center is a large urban institution located
on the fringes of a New York City ghetto. Since it is one of the only
voluntary hospitals in the metropolitan area that has a child psychiatry
inpatient unit, patients come from all parts of New York City and its
environs for treatment. Many of the children (maximum capacity 15)
are economically and culturally deprived. All are severely troubled and
have troubled families. The children may be as young as 4 years and
as old as 13 or 14. Most are in middle latency. Most have problems
with aggression, low frustration tolerance, and impulsivity. About
one-third can be classified as schizophrenic or schizotypal (DSM III)
and one-third as having severe behavior or conduct disturbances.
Many are significantly depressed and many have attention-deficit
disorders, language disorders, and learning disorders.

The aim of this book is to describe the approach on this short-term
(3 weeks to 3 months) child psychiatry unit. A medical model is
followed in terms of a stepwise process: There is an assessment of the
child and family, a diagnosis (in the broad sense) is arrived at, and
a treatment plan is formulated and implemented. The evaluation,
diagnosis, and treatment of each child proceed within a psychodynamic
and developmental frame of reference. This process is accomplished
via the integration of data from the staff, who are organized into a
team structure using principles derived from therapeutic communities.
Evaluation and treatment is thus accomplished not by one or two
individuals but by a group of people working conjointly with the child
and family.

A milieu that attempts to evaluate and treat a group of severely
disturbed children cannot be static. There is constant dynamic interplay
among the staff, between staff and children, and among the children
themselves. The resultant of these various forces is dependent on the
factors operative at the time. These factors include the pathology and
level of development of the group of children living on the unit at the
time; the pathology of the families of these children; external factors
such as holidays, vacations, and unforeseen events; and most importantly,
interactions among the staff.

The chapters in this volume have been written by the people who
have firsthand knowledge of the treatment of these hospitalized children.
The various components of the evaluation and treatment process described
frequently change because of the very dynamic nature of the unit,
yet the underlying principles remain the same.

Leon Hoffman, M.D.

---

*Berlin, I.N. (1978). Developmental issues in the psychiatric hospitaliza-
tion of children. *Am. J. Psychiatry 135:* 1044-1048.

CONTRIBUTORS

ROBYN ABRAMSON, M.A., O.T.R.,
Occupational Therapy Supervisor,
Child and Adolescent Services,
Mount Sinai Medical Center,
New York, New York

ROBERT M. BERK, M.D.,
Pediatric Liaison,
Inpatient Unit,
Senior Clinical Instructor,
Mount Sinai School of Medicine,
New York, New York

ARNOLD COHEN, M.D.,
Assistant Clinical Professor,
Mount Sinai School of Medicine,
New York, New York

NORMAN A. FRIEDMAN, M.S.,
Administrator, P.S. 106,
Mount Sinai Medical Center,
New York, New York

LEON HOFFMAN, M.D.,
Psychiatrist-In-Charge,
Inpatient Unit,
Assistant Clinical Professor,
Mount Sinai School of Medicine,
New York, New York

CHRISTINE JOHNS, B.S.N., M.S.,
Senior Clinical Nurse/Coordinator,
Day Treatment Program,
Mount Sinai Medical Center,
New York, New York

JESSICA HELLINGER-KASLICK,
 M.S.W., C.S.W.,
Department of Social Work Service,
Mount Sinai Medical Center,
New York, New York

PAUL KENNEDY, M.D.,
Clinical Instructor,
Mount Sinai School of Medicine,
New York, New York

RONALD RAWITT, M.D.,
Clinical Instructor,
Mount Sinai School of Medicine,
New York, New York

MARY REHILL, B.S., R.N.,
Clinical Supervisor, Nursing,
Child and Adolescent Services,
Mount Sinai Medical Center,
New York, New York

LOIS SHEIN, M.S.W., C.S.W.,
Social Work Supervisor in Child
 Psychiatry,
Mount Sinai Medical Center,
New York, New York

ELAINE SIMON, O.T.R.,
Occupational Therapist,
Day Treatment Program,
Mount Sinai Medical Center,
New York, New York

MARSHA SILVERTON, M.S.W.,
 C.S.W.,
Department of Social Work Service,
Mount Sinai Medical Center,
New York, New York

MARY ANN WAGNER, R.N.,
Senior Clinical Nurse,
Child Psychiatry,
Inpatient Unit,
Mount Sinai Medical Center,
New York, New York

CONTENTS

Chapter 1

AN HISTORICAL OVERVIEW OF MILIEU THERAPY

Leon Hoffman

The term "milieu therapy" was coined in Germany in the early 1900s to describe a new hospital treatment for psychiatric patients. It was first called *activere behandlugen*–more active therapy–and later, *milieu therapie*. Its main element was the active role taken by the nursing staff in working with patients. A forerunner of this type of treatment was "moral treatment", developed at the end of the eighteenth century. This marked the beginning of kindly and humane treatment for psychiatric patients. Its founder, P. Pinel, created a revolution in his time by urging that the mentally ill be treated compassionately and with understanding.

In the late 1800s, in the United States Dorothea Dix championed the establishment of large rural institutions (state hospitals) for the purpose of administering moral treatment to psychiatric patients. After a brief successful period, this program failed for several reasons. The hospitals became more concerned with administration and control rather than with therapy. The psychiatrists of the time had a neuropathological approach, that is, they were more concerned with diagnosis and prognosis than with treatment. Furthermore, the majority of patients in state hospitals were "foreign insane paupers" who were not good candidates for moral treatment because they did not speak English (Almond, 1974).

In the 1920s and 1930s H.S. Sullivan stressed the role of the environment in the treatment of schizophrenics. Thus the concept of "total push therapy" was developed where the entire ward staff was considered important in the treatment of the patient. The term milieu therapy became the all-embracing phrase for these techniques. At this time the Menningers developed their program in which the therapist prescribed to the ward staff the desired type of social interaction that should take place with patients, on the basis of the psychotherapy data collected on them. Chestnut Lodge and Austin Riggs developed similar approaches (Almond, 1974).

A somewhat different orientation to the hospital treatment of psychiatric patients evolved from the concept of therapeutic community (Jones, 1953). In the therapeutic community the decision-making process includes all staff members and patients, not solely the psychotherapist. The emphasis is on group therapy, and individual therapy is minimized or restricted to a supportive role.

The nature of the groups and activities in a therapeutic community depend on the types of patients on the ward as well as the interests and capabilities of the staff. A central meeting is the "community meeting" or "patient-staff" meeting with everyone present. The "culture" of the community is conveyed and reinforced at this meeting. This meeting is reflective of both the unity and coherence as well as the disorganization among patients and staff, and is therefore a good indicator of the therapeutic status of the community.

The second central characteristic of a therapeutic community is the importance placed on the role definition of both patients and staff. In large state hospitals, aides make most decisions about the patient but must attribute these to higher authority. By contrast, in the therapeutic community the aide is brought into the decision-making process where he or she shares that responsibility with the other staff. The role of the nurse is shifted from passive implementer of medical orders to active therapeutic agent. The role of the senior personnel is seen less as that of medical professionals and therapists and more as educators and role models. Patients are viewed as actors, initiators, collaborators, and managers of their own affairs (Almond, 1974).

These basic theoretical concepts of milieu therapy and therapeutic community are applicable to the types of treatments children receive in psychiatric hospitals or residential treatment centers (Barker, 1974).

The first children's psychiatric units were opened in the 1920s. The Bellevue Hospital Children's Ward was originally organized in order to treat children with behavior disorders secondary to the epidemic of encephalitis lethargica. In 1924, Kings Park Hospital began to treat many of these children. The Child's Guidance Home in Cincinnati and the Franklin School in Philadelphia were two other early centers. Prior to this time the only children's facilities were orphanages. Some extremely disturbed children were admitted to adult psychiatric wards. During the 1920s and 1930s, as public assistance increased, children who were formerly sent to orphanages remained at home. This shift was accelerated by the findings of the detrimental effect of affective deprivation in large institutions. Thus, a shift ensued in the focus of child-care institutions: From providing shelter for homeless children to treating children with emotional problems. For example, Hawthorne, which had been founded in 1906 to treat homeless Jewish delinquents, was providing individual psychotherapy by the 1930s (American Psychiatric Association, 1957; Evangelakis, 1974).

The most influential forces in child care at this time were the child guidance movement and psychoanalytic psychology. Many residential treatment centers included the use of psychiatrists, social workers, and psychologists in their classical roles. Aichhorn (1935) was the first to apply psychoanalytic principles in residential treatment of children. He recognized that the effects of peer relationships and transference feelings toward the counselors could be used therapeutically. Many of the residential treatment centers were then organized in order to provide a benign environment as a support for a psychoanalytically oriented psychotherapy. Most of the literature about residential treatment in hospital and nonhospital settings has been grounded on ego psychological concepts (Bettleheim, 1950, 1966; Noshpitz, 1962; Redl, 1959a,b). Much of the current literatures stresses the application of behavioral principles, developmental and educational principles (Whittaker and Trieschman, 1972), community work, and medication. Currently, there is tremendous debate over institutional versus community treatment because it has been shown that a crucial variable in determining outcome is the child's post-treatment environment (Whittaker, 1975).

Two of the earliest and best of the detailed descriptions of children's psychiatric wards are from the 1930s. The papers by Potter (1935) from Psychiatric Institute and by Bender (1937) from Bellevue Hospital detail specific operating principles which are still applicable at the present time.

Potter states that a child may require hospitalization for several reasons: (1) for diagnostic purposes if a physical condition is thought to be the underlying problem; (2) in young children, to differentiate low intelligence from emotional problems; (3) to determine whether a behavior problem is the result of an organic defect or a result of spoiling; (4) because of the need for a controlled environment; (5) because more treatment is needed than can be given as an outpatient; (6) because a difficult home situation necessitates a vacation for both child and family; (7) treatment would more readily be initiated in the hospital; and (8) in certain cases a period of hospital treatment is needed prior to boarding home placement. It is striking how these indications for admission are similar to those in use today (Silver, 1976). Further, Potter states that the manner of admission is very important. Both the child and parents need to be taken into confidence before admission can be arranged successfully. We have seen over and over how important a factor this is. For example, a parent who is ambivalent about a child's hospitalization can easily sabotage any positive gains made by the child.

In describing the staffing of an inpatient unit, Potter emphasizes that the individual patient's contact with nurses, occupational therapists, teachers, psychologists, social workers, and psychiatrists is of utmost therapeutic value. He stresses the types of personalities these professionals need to have. Vital character traits include a real interest in children, a sense of humor, enthusiasm, patience, and objectivity. Staff are essentially parent-surrogates. Potter also stresses the importance of working with families to try to "modify faulty attitudes" of the parents. He emphasizes the use of psychotherapy, and especially, the importance of establishing a rapport with the child. He discusses in great detail the problem of discipline and advocates the use of isolation, that is, what is now referred to as "time-out," as the only effective active disciplinary measure.

In contrast to Potter, Bender emphasizes ward group activities rather than individual contact. She states that this is done because of (1) a lack of trained psychiatrists, (2) it is a more successful means of talking and communicating with children and getting them to express their problems, and (3) there is a definite value of group therapy in aiding in the socialization of children. However, it should be noted that the ward at Bellevue that Bender discusses in her work was a short-term ward with an average stay of 30 days. There were approximately three to four admissions and discharges per day and many of the children were rehospitalized two or three times.

Bender states that a children's ward has to satisfy all of the child's needs for physical growth and health and for exercising the child's expanding physical, intellectual, emotional, and social functions. There needs to be free expression of neurotic complexes to the psychiatrist. The child should feel relief from feelings of anxiety, guilt, inferiority, and insecurity and should receive demonstrations of affection and approval from the adults. In addition, the child should be able to express both feelings of affection and impulses of aggression. There need to be opportunities for the child to become socially at ease and acceptable to others and there should be an attempt at crystallization of those ideologies of the child which are suitable for both the child and

the surrounding social milieu in which he or she lives. All of these
goals appear to be idealistic and difficult to envision as occurring in a
30-day hospitalization.

Bender, as well as Potter, stresses the importance of staff conferences
for communication and sharing of data by all staff. Bender also
recommends the use of time-out procedures for disruptive behavior.
In addition, Bender warns that serious difficulties in the group may
result from the uncontrolled behavior of a "seriously neurotic child" or
"organically psychotic child." The only effective remedy may be to
remove that child from the group.

Bender also describes a whole range of group activities: play groups,
discussion groups, art groups, music projects, puppet projects, and
spontaneous groups. She also describes group treatment in staff
conferences, which is similar to the technique described by Redl (1959a),
and known as "the life space interview."

Fritz Redl has provided both a theoretical basis as well as practical
instructions for working with children in residential settings. He
details many specific elements, as follows (Redl, 1959b):

> 1. Social structure: A hospital unit or residential
> center is more like a harem society than a family.
> Its closest relative is that of a summer camp in
> which there are many adults supervising and taking
> care of the children. In such a setting, the role
> distribution of the various staff members must be
> clear to the children. Pecking orders invariably
> occur both among the children and the adults and
> the children can tell whom they can approach for
> what and who has more authority than whom.

> 2. The children can intuitively tell what values
> the staff regards as most important no matter
> what is written down on paper. Each center has
> its own climate. However, both Redl and Caudill
> (American Psychiatric Association, 1957) state
> that research is needed in order to be able to
> describe the climate so that one can do research
> as to which climate is more therapeutic for a
> particular group of children.

> 3. The climate prevalent in a given institution
> influences directly the routines, rituals, and
> behavioral regulations which are in effect in that
> particular setting. Redl emphasizes that there
> is no data available on the clinical relevance of
> whatever specific practice may be in vogue in
> any particular place. For example, even though
> there is a general routine set-up, the particular
> mix of activities depends on the particular group
> of people working that day as well as the particular
> mix of children.

> 4. The impact of the group process on a particular
> child may be very difficult to assess. Any group
> of children reacts quite differently from their
> behavior in individual relationships. In groups
> there may be contagion chains, scapegoat formations,
> mascot cultivations, status struggles, spontaneous
> group discipline, and disorganization. Questions

about group life include what should be the balance between isolation and privacy and group experience. Some children cannot be exposed to group life. In a group living situation the individual children affect each other by their actions in an accentuated way because of close and constant contact. This is especially so in a small closed unit such as the one at Mount Sinai.

5. Perhaps the most important milieu factor is the attitudes and feelings of the staff. For example, punishment from a benign adult may convey the implication that the child is still loved. Related to this is the degree of behavioral disturbance the adult can tolerate from the children towards himself. As Redl states so aptly, "One simply can't stand more than 1/2 pound spittle in the face a day, professional attitude or no."

6. The structure and content of games and activities has an important overall effect on the children. For example, a game that is too stimulating would be inappropriate before bedtime. Or, if one builds a safety zone in a game, it allows a child to withdraw without having to admit he's tired or scared.

7. In addition to the actual activity, the space, equipment, time factor, and props deserve serious consideration. Redl states that in hospitals, psychiatrists and sociologists may ignore these factors when studying group process, whereas nurses and attendants have learned by bitter experience how important these factors are. For example, one may invite disaster if one allows a baseball to be thrown during quiet time. We have come to understand how important a consideration that is, particularly because our available space on the unit is limited. When there's a particular mix of children who stimulate or provoke each other, free play with balls, for example, may lead to chaos.

8. Events that occur outside of the unit have an effect on the children. Visitors to the unit as well as excursions or home visits have a tremendous effect not only on the individual children involved but on all the children. On our unit we have seen the behavioral effects of the ambivalences and anxieties about home visits and a parent who comes and yells at the child or at the staff. Much anxiety is generated by such occurrences and many children inevitably manifest their anxiety by behavioral disturbances.

In a hospital setting, another anxiety-provoking situation is seeing sick patients from other wards. This may lead to fears such as "Why am I here?" and "Am I going to get an operation?" Our ward's

location across from the neoplastic unit has
occasionally led to anxiety on both the children's
and staff's part in seeing very ill patients as
well as metal coffins.

9. A role for the staff in many situations is to
try to be a buffer between the child and the
effects of the environment (both outside and
inside). One technique that Redl recommends
is the life space interview, which is detailed later.

10. Finally, the staff has to have enough clinical
resiliency to vary between flexibility and rigidity.
When there's danger of impulse-panic, behavioral
controls must increase—"tighten up." In the early
phases of treatment and when rampant pathology
is evident, more controls are necessary than later
on in treatment. On a short-term unit with the
recurrent apprehensions generated by admissions
and discharges, behavioral controls and limits to
one degree or another are almost always mandatory.

Redl lists several ways in which a milieu can be therapeutic. The
most important one is that the milieu needs to be free from any counter-
therapeutic agents, such as cruel punishments. Obviously, basic needs
such as eating have to be met. Activities have to be based on an
awareness of developmental and cultural considerations. For example,
a timid middle-class child needs to be approached differently from a
"toughie." The milieu needs to have rules and regulations, but there
are points where the inability to make exceptions becomes untherapeutic.
Very importantly, a milieu provides new models for identification.

In fact, many residential centers which do not have specific therapy
programs attribute their successes to the new and stable identifications
the children are able to make (Noshpitz, 1962).

Redl warns that there's no such thing as *the* therapeutic milieu.
The character of the milieu and, as a result, its therapeutic effectiveness
or ineffectiveness, depends on the staff, their values, and how they
carry them out. One cannot say that a milieu can be automatically
created by carefully orchestrating all activities, nor can one say that
all that is needed for a good treatment milieu is a "milieu-convinced
ward boss to make his nurses feel comfortable and to hold a few gripe
sessions." Both approaches are too simplistic. Very importantly, the
treatment goals determine what is therapeutic for any particular child.

There are four patterns that describe the place of milieu therapy
in the total treatment plan in any individual treatment center (American
Psychiatric Association, 1957).

1. The first is one in which the primary emphasis is
on the clear structuring of the child's living experience
and on striving to provide the optimal opportunity for
gratification through activities and interpersonal
relationships (Whittaker, 1975). Some centers operate
under this concept because of a conviction that it is
the most therapeutic approach, whereas others do so
because they are unable to provide psychotherapy.
Certain children whose difficulties arise from deprived
and disorganized backgrounds improve with milieu
therapy, and then neurotic symptoms appear which
would be amenable to psychotherapy.

2. A second approach involves an equal emphasis on psychotherapy and milieu therapy.

3. A third approach is one in which the only purpose is to have the child in a setting which enhances his capacity to utilize individual therapy.

4. The fourth approach is similar to the third, that is, the psychotherapy is of prime importance. However, there is a more conscious attempt in the milieu for re-education (this term being used not in a cognitive sense). There is permission for regression on the assumption that the child will regress to the developmental phase of which he was unable to master normal conflicts and then he will have a corrective experience with the staff. This approach is a long-term one that requires close integration between the child care staff and the psychotherapists. An essential element in this collaboration is an acceptance of one's task and a lack of competitiveness. This is the approach of Bettleheim and Sylvester (1948). This plan allows the child to gradually internalize controls with a minimal of external rules. One-to-one relationships with various staff members allow the child to experience gratifications that he has never had.

The next chapter details the philosophy of the milieu on the Child Psychiatry Inpatient Unit at the Mount Sinai Medical Center, the remainder of the book details various aspects of the program.

REFERENCES

Aichorn, A. (1935). *Wayward Youth*. New York: Viking

Almond, R. (1974). *The Healing Community*. New York: Jason Aronson Inc.

American Psychiatric Association (1957). *Psychiatric Inpatient Treatment of Children*. Baltimore: Lord Baltimore.

Barker, P. (1974). *The Residential Psychiatric Treatment of Children*. New York: Wiley and Sons.

Bender, L. (1937). Group activities on a children's ward as methods of psychotherapy. *Am. J. Psychiatry 93:* 1151-1173.

Bettleheim, B. (1950). *Love is Not Enough*. Glencoe, Ill: The Free Press.

Bettleheim, B. (1966). Training the child care worker in a residential center. *Am. J. Orthopsychiatry 36:* 694-705.

Bettleheim, B., and Sylvester, E. (1948). A therapeutic milieu. *Am. J. Orthopsychiatry 18:* 191-206.

Evangelakis, M. (1974). *A Manual for Residential and Day Treatment of Children*. Springfield, Ill.: Charles C Thomas.

Jones, M. (1953). *The Therapeutic Community: A New Treatment Method in Psychiatry*. New York: Basic Books.

Noshpitz, J. (1962). Notes on the theory of residential treatment. *J. Am. Acad. Child Psychiatry 1:* 284-296.

Potter, H. (1935). The treatment of problem children in a psychiatric hospital. *Am. J. Psychiatry 91:* 869-880.

Redl, F. (1959a). Life space interview techniques. *Am. J. Orthopsychiatry 29:* 1-28.

Redl, F. (1959b). The concept of a therapeutic milieu. *Am. J. Orthopsychiatry 29:* 721-736.

Silver, L.B., ed. (1976). *Professional Standards Review Organizations: A Handbook for Child Psychiatrists*. Washington, D.C.: American Academy of Child Psychiatry.

Whittaker, J. (1975). The ecology of child treatment: A developmental educational approach to the therapeutic milieu. *J. Aut. Childh. Schiz.* 5:223-237.

Whittaker, J., and Trieschman, A., eds. (1972). *Children Away From Home: A Source Book in Residential Treatment*. Chicago: Aldine.

Chapter 2

PHILOSOPHY OF THE MILIEU

Leon Hoffman

Over the past 10 years there has been a gradual change on the Child Psychiatry Inpatient Unit at the Mount Sinai Medical Center. Kleinberger (1966) stated that during the 3-month stay "there is intensive therapeutic contact in both individual and milieu areas as well as intervention in family dynamics through weekly casework contact with the parents." The nurse was considered the "mother-surrogate" for the children (Blau and Slaff, 1964). During this period of time the psychotherapists were the child psychiatry fellows supervised by attending child psychiatrists who were not involved in the day-to-day treatment of the child on the ward. There were no lay therapists and the social workers did "casework" in which "the treatment of the adult is carefully kept child centered " (Blau and Slaff, 1964).

Clearly, the emphasis of the milieu was to support the child for the work in psychotherapy. There were, however, many children for whom the relationships with the staff with whom they spent "their other 23 hours" were more important than the relationship with their therapist. For these children identification with these new, relatively stable objects was the most therapeutic element of their ward stay. The ward itself was often seen as a safe haven. Safirstein's (1967) concept of institutional transference aptly applies. Many children would come back to visit and ask about the whereabouts of particular staff and children who were in the hospital at the time of their stay on the ward. For example, one child visited after several years and asked, "Who is sleeping in *my* bed now?"

Two major changes have occurred which have altered the view of the functions of the milieu: (1) the marked change in the character of the patient population, and (2) the introduction of other mental health workers as therapists, the development of a team approach, the strengthening of family orientation, and a much sharper definition of staff functions within the milieu.

Kleinberger (1966) described the first 100 children admitted to the unit. Seventy-two of the children were white; 13 black and 15, Puerto Rican. Of the white children, only one came from a low socioeconomic background, whereas 10 black children and 12 Puerto Rican children came from such a background. There was a selectivity in the type of children admitted, that is, "if it was felt that the degree of psychopathology would not make long term residential care an obvious necessity,

9

and if the child could be handled in this metropolitan general hospital setting."

In contrast, recent ethnic proportions consist of one-third to one-half white children, the remainder being black, Puerto Rican, or of mixed parentage. Of all the children, 75 percent are from classes 4 or 5 (Hollingshead and Redlich, 1958), the lower socioeconomic groups. The majority of these children are hospitalized on Medicaid. The length of stay is usually limited to 3 months for the children on Medicaid, white middle-class children, that is, those with Blue Cross coverage, can be hospitalized for only 21 or 30 days.

Our experience has been similar to others (Whittaker, 1975), that the population of children in residential and day treatment seems much sicker than just a few years ago. Whittaker describes a symptom cluster which he labels "the empty bucket syndrome" (a colloquialism commonly used by many psychiatrists). The characteristic problems of these children are:

1. Poorly developed impulse control
2. Low self-image
3. Poorly developed modulation of emotion
4. Relationship deficits
5. Family pain and strain
6. Special learning disabilities
7. Limited play skills

These children, as well as their families, are very difficult to treat. They require an extraordinary amount of input, effort, and structure from the staff. They come to the hospital most commonly because someone in the child's environment, that is, parent, school, agency, therapist, etc., has decided that the child's symptoms and behavior are so problematic that they cannot be treated with outpatient care. Outpatient evaluation and treatment of one kind or other may have been unsuccessfully attempted, but often none has been tried. At times a family crisis precipitates a suicidal or aggressive gesture on the part of the child which results in admission to the unit. At other times a child who is acutely suicidal or grossly psychotic needs rapid admission. Most often, however, the decision to hospitalize the child is the result of the judgment that a period away from the stresses of the environment will provide a clearer picture of the child's strengths and pathology, and begin a treatment process for both the child and the family. During the time in the hospital a structure is provided in which both the child and parent(s) are evaluated and engaged in therapeutic interactions with various staff members. This period is most importantly used to decide the best long-term disposition of the child. About 50 percent of the children go on to long-term residential treatment centers.

The ward utilizes a psychodynamic and developmental frame of reference within a medical model in order to understand and evaluate the child and his or her family and to implement appropriate plans. Behavior modification techniques and medication are used when indicated.

There are four steps in the course of hospitalization. First, the child and family are helped to establish relationships with the staff and other children and to develop an adequate working alliance to enable the evaluating and treatment process to begin. At times, the major effort during this period includes intensive work with the parents who may feel guilty, anxious, and ambivalent about hospitalizing their child. These feelings often lead them to project their guilt onto the staff. The staff has to deal with the parents' various defensive maneuvers therapeutically and avoid counterdefensiveness.

Second, the assessment of the child and his family begins during the early phase of hospitalization. The source of conflicts as well as the depth of both the child's and parents' psychopathology is determined both in individual and group sessions. Formal psychological, sensori-motor, cognitive, and educational batteries are administered. Neurological, speech and hearing, and pediatric consultations are obtained when needed. Most importantly, the ward, where the child lives, provides an arena for ongoing evaluation of his relationship to the other children, to the adults on the ward, and to his parents. The staff observes the areas in which the child is competent or excels as well as the areas in which he exhibits problems. His or her fantasy life is explored via art therapy and individual psychotherapy. The staff must be keen observers of behavior in order to define the problem areas.

Third, specific treatment plans are implemented during the hospital stay. The specific plans occur within the structure of the milieu as defined below. Fourth, and often a very difficult step, is defining and implementing an adequate posthospital disposition given the limitation of real possibilities.

The team concept is the most efficacious organizational structure to deal with the complex problems of the children and their families. Historically, both residential treatment centers for children and adult psychiatric hospitals have often experienced severe conflicts between the caretakers and the psychotherapists. These conflicts may arise out of unresolved issues of status and role functions. "Whose job is more important and more effective?" Brunstetter (1969) states that it has been "unseemly in recent years for workers to express openly feelings about status (because it is) considered childish." Such feelings often remain underground, unresolved, and affect the treatment of the child. These feelings of lack of status are accentuated whenever a co-worker feels that his or her ideas and suggestions have been ignored. With a team approach the members of the team gradually come to feel that even if their point of view is not implemented, at least it is considered seriously. This process thus can help eliminate the very common confusion between being ignored and not agreeing.

Maxwell Jones (1968) discusses in depth the decision-making process in a therapeutic community. The entire process is a difficult one because the concept of consensus is involved. Even though one person usually has ultimate authority, he or she cannot make decisions without at least the consent of a majority of the group. In fact, Jones comments that leadership roles may be shared and rotated. Hidden agendas, problem on feedback and spread of rumors are important issues that need to be brought out into the open.

There has to be intensive cooperation and teamwork of the staff in any active milieu working with severely disturbed children. Whether there is mutual collaboration or undercutting of each other's roles depends upon the interrelationships among the various staff members. Under the old model, where there was a dramatic distinction between psychotherapy and everything else, roles were clearly spelled out and there was a clear-cut demarcation of functions.

Very clearly, such a model leads to one set of problems and conflicts. As the model has changed and continues to evolve there is a resultant potential for greater satisfaction as well as potential for a different set of problems and conflicts.

The greater satisfaction obviously has to do with all members of the staff feeling and being more actively involved in the treatment of the child. In this way, their professional growth is enhanced. The area of potential conflicts lies in the sphere of intrastaff relations. In addition

to the issues of status and function, a major source of potential conflict
lies in the area of role specificity and role diffusion. The "ideal"
therapeutic community favors a pervasive diffusion of roles. In a
classical psychotherapy hospital there is clear delineation of specific
roles and functions. The unit at Mount Sinai is formulated on what
might be seen as an amalgamation of these two concepts.

This approach to ward treatment, when implemented correctly, blurs
the clear-cut distinctions between individual psychotherapy, group psychotherapy, and milieu therapy. Noshpitz (1962) organized his unit
whereby the psychiatrist saw the child in individual sessions only when
necessary, and then around specific issues. On the unit at Mount Sinai,
each child has a primary therapist whose function is to (1) integrate
the data from all the various disciplines, (2) establish a special relationship with the child and his family, (3) begin to understand the child's
and family's mental life, and (4) help other staff members understand
the child's behavior in terms of the child's psychodynamics in order to
provide for more rational forms of interventions during day-to-day
treatment (Berlin and Christ, 1969).

Children who have internalized neurotic conflicts often do better
with a differentiation between their psychotherapy and the day-to-day
management of their daily life activities (psychotherapy-administrator
split). The population at Mount Sinai mainly consists of children with
severe ego developmental arrests with diminished capacity for abstract
thinking and maintenance of object relationships. These disturbances
permeate their entire character structure and therefore the treatment
has to be based on a foundation of need satisfaction. For these children
a psychotherapist-administrator-caretaker combination is preferred
(Harrison, McDermott, and Chethik, 1969). The therapist is a giving
person, helps in setting limits, and helps the child gain insight into
his or her problems. On the unit, the child psychiatry fellows and
the social workers are involved in both individual psychotherapy as well
as in the group and milieu aspects of the program.

The child guidance model of a social worker seeing the family and
the psychiatrist seeing the child is not appropriate for a short-term
inpatient program. The treatment needs to be family-centered and,
with rare exceptions, the child's therapist is the one in regular contact
with the family. Long-standing biases, however, are so incorporated
into staff attitudes that one occasionally hears such statements as "the
child is just here for milieu, he's not getting any treatment" or "he's a
management problem." Both these statements imply that the treatment
the child receives within the milieu is secondary to the individual psychotherapy. The chart records are also an issue because insurance
companies do not reimburse for "milieu therapy" on the grounds that
such treatment is not properly medical but merely custodial.

Noshpitz (1962) has detailed how his model of milieu therapy, in
fact, is very active treatment and very distinct from benign custodial
care. This active milieu model is the basis for many of the techniques
implemented on the unit at Mount Sinai.

The two elements of this model, ego support and ego interpretation,
derive from Redl's (1959) concept of the "life space interview techniques."
Redl uses the terms "emotional first aid on the spot" (ego support) and
the "clinical exploitation of Life's events" (ego interpretation). Both
of these techniques require an informed staff and continual staff training
through discussions, because the "common sense approach of well-intentioned
but nontrained people may not work" (Noshpitz, 1962). Both techniques
require an "on the spot diagnosis" (Redl, 1959) by the particular
staff member in order to decide what is the best approach to the particular

child in the particular situation. Careful observations of the child's behavior is required in order for all staff members to integrate the data, decide what elements are playing a role in the child's relationships to the various staff members, and to formulate a consistent staff approach.

The term "ego support" implies a group of treatment tactics aimed at strengthening, consolidating, and giving sharper outline to an ego that lacks the type of integrity that should have come with normal development. Examples of this tactic include limiting aggressive behavior, anticipating situations that might overwhelm the children, rapidly moving in when early signs of disorganization occur, and deciding what is the appropriate degree of isolation, comfort, containment, and control that is required.

Ego interpretation is a strategy in which the staff delicately interprets the defensive aspect of behavior while controlling overt "acting out." The essence of this approach requires an understanding of the meaning of the behavior and attempting to interpret to the child its underlying significance, for example, interpreting to the child his underlying anxiety when he begins to hit out (if this is the case).

It is abundantly clear that this approach can be both inordinately difficult but at the same time quite rewarding. The difficulties lie in the fact that a "cookbook" cannot be written. Redl and Wineman (1951) detail innumerable clinical examples of behaviors and appropriate interventions. However, each situation is different and many factors have to be taken into consideration in order to determine the best approach at a particular time.

Thus, even though certain staff members have the expertise and responsibility to carry out specific functions, there are many areas in which there is an overlap in function. The conflicts with which a child is struggling in his individual sessions will affect his behavior in the program with the occupational and art therapist, with his teacher in school, and with his nurse during activities of daily living. Each staff member fosters the child's developmental progression via age-appropriate and developmentally appropriate tasks and goals. In addition, the staff needs to be aware of the conflicts and stresses (intrapsychic, interpersonal, and familial) that may interfere with the child's performance in order to determine whether "ego support: or "ego interpretation" is the appropriate techniques and respond as effectively as possible.

A clinical illustration: Patient M. is an 11-year-old black preadolescent girl. Her life began as the 3-lb baby born to a mother who was herself abused and rejected. M.'s life was filled with multiple rejections, foster placements, prior residential treatment, and many instances of suspected, but legally unproven, abuse. She was admitted because of a history of running away, not obeying, screaming, yelling, and fighting. A goal of hospitalization was to prepare for her long-term residential treatment. She was negativistic and clearly depressed on admission; she could think of no one to be with if she had to go to a desert island. Her mother, with a history of maternal rejection, child abuse, and many foster placements, had in turn completely rejected M. She was in treatment with a diagnosis of adult MBD with a drug-dependency problem. M.'s father, a reformed drug addict, became interested in M. and attended family meetings.

M.'s affect hunger, which she experienced as an endless search for a good feeding object, was probably the underlying dynamic for her symptom of running away. It was poignantly demonstrated by her coming to visit the unit between the day of her screening and her admission 1 week later.

The major goal in a short-term unit with such a child is to help her begin to trust adults since past experience with adults has taught her the opposite. It would, of course, be naive or grandiose to think that a 3-month stay might have an enduring and strong impact on a child like M. On the other hand, it would be nihilistic to adopt the attitude of "What's the point of doing anything?" A 3-month stay can indeed have a significant effect on a child, even one as deprived as M.

First, a milieu approach with many different adults working together is necessary because someone like M. cannot tolerate the intensity of a one-to-one relationship. Second, the treatment of such a severely aggressive and abusive child cannot remain in the hands of one or two people because of the counterreactions and countertransferences elicited. No matter how well analyzed one may be, it would not be too difficult to become enraged at M.'s provocativeness or be frightened of her aggressive outbursts.

Because of this, simply a supportive orientation, in essence saying to M., "Look, the staff is here to help," cannot work. Long before she could hear that, she would have alienated virtually every staff member who would then be clamoring for her discharge to "a more appropriate unit." In fact, in cases such as these the staff simply becomes another set of rejecting adults. M. repeatedly pushed staff away, perhaps even more so when they showed interest.

A behavior modification program integrated with dynamic techniques was instituted on the premise that aggressive adolescents often respond to the structure and limits of a "program" more effectively because the struggle with the adult authority figure is avoided and displaced onto an impersonal agent. In essence, the adult says, "I'm not telling you to do this, the program is" (Rossman and Knesper, 1976).

This technique may be viewed, according to Noshpitz's categories, as "ego support."

Difficulties ensued around the implementation of the program because many staff were in disagreement about its use. In fact, a difficult patient can split the staff, eliciting all kinds of counterreactions. Small ad hoc meetings, in addition to regular conferences, were held in order to try to alleviate and prevent some of these staff problems.

The "ego interpretation" technique was used both by the child's primary therapist as well as by other members. The major thrust of the interpretation was: "M. pushed people away in the same way she felt pushed out by her mother." At the same time the staff kept coming back consistently, even though M. rejected them.

Despite the staff conflicts, the plan seemed to work: M. was seeking out more staff and showing improvement in the intensity and frequency of her aggressive outbursts; she began to seek out sessions with her therapist rather than reject him; she verbalized her feeling that there is no one to take care of her. Ideally, of course, M. should stay on the same unit for a very long time and gradually return to some non-institutional environment. However, her short-term hospital treatment allowed M. to become more integrated and enabled her to be placed in a long-term treatment facility.

It is of interest to compare the difference between the milieu at Mount Sinai and that planned on a developmental/educational paradigm (Whittaker, 1975). The latter milieu relies mainly on ego-supportive and ego-building techniques. The milieu at Mount Sinai also provides this in a variety of ways. The school, with its individual tutorial program, is a nonpressured environment where the child starts at the level he is presently at and progresses at his own rate. The therapeutic activities program complements this by providing for each child individually in order to develop his cognitive and social skills. The nursing staff supports the child, helps his social skills, and provides for new models of identification. In addition, however, the use of the method of ego interpretation provides another special and very valuable tool. Even in short-term treatment it promotes ego development and progression by enabling the child to gain some insight and control over some of his instinctual urges. The remainder of this book details the implementation of this point of view.

REFERENCES

Abramson, R., Hoffman, L., and Johns, C. (1979). Play group for early latency age children on a short term psychiatric unit. *Int. J. Group Psychother.* in press.

Berlin, I.N., and Christ, A. (1969). The unique role of the child psychiatry trainee on an inpatient or day care unit. *J. Am. Acad. Child Psychiatry 8:*247-258.

Blau, A., and Slaff, B. (1964). Child psychiatry division in a general hospital. *N.Y. State J. Med. 64:*1096-1100.

Brunstetter, R. (1969). Status, role and the function of supervision in the residential treatment center for children. *J. Am. Acad. Child Psychiatry 8:*259-271.

Harrison, S., McDermott, J., and Chethik, M. (1969). Residential treatment of children: The psychotherapist-administrator. *J. Am. Acad. Child Psychiatry 8:*385-410.

Hollinghead, A., and Redlich, F. (1958). *Social Class and Mental Illness.* New York: John Wiley and Son.

Jones, M. (1968). *Beyond the Therapeutic Community: Social Learning and Social Psychiatry.* New Haven: Yale Univ. Press.

Kleinberger, E. (1966). Hallucinations in children. Unpublished.

Noshpitz, J. (1962). Notes on the theory of residential treatment. *J. Am. Acad. Child Psychiatry 1:*284-296.

Redl, F. (1959). Life space interview techniques. *Am. J. Orthopsychiatry 29:*1-28.

Rossman, P., and Knesper, D. (1976). The early phase of hospital treatment for disruptive adolescents: the integration of behavioral and dynamic techniques. *J. Am. Acad. Child Psychiatry 15:*693-708.

Safirstein, S. (1967). Institutional transference. *Psych. Quart.* July: 1-10.

Tucker, G., and Maxmen, J. (1973). The practice of hospital psychiatry: A formulation. *Am. J. Psychiatry 130:*887-891.

Whittaker, J. (1975). The ecology of child treatment: A developmental educational approach to the therapeutic milieu. *J. Aut. Childh. Schiz. 5:*223-237.

Chapter 3

CRITERIA FOR ADMISSION AND INTAKE PROCESS

Leon Hoffman

Criteria for admission into a child psychiatry inpatient unit often are not as clear cut as those for an adult psychiatric unit. Social factors plus the severity of the child's symptoms need to be considered in order to decide whether or not inpatient treatment is warranted (Silver, 1976, p. 26). Most children are referred for inpatient treatment "not because they are suffering from some particular disorder, but because the people in their immediate environment (parents, teachers, therapist, police, etc.) either cannot or will not continue to tolerate the behavior" (Sackin and Meyer, 1976).

Children referred to the Mount Sinai Medical Center Child Psychiatry Inpatient Unit come from the outpatient department, social agencies, schools, other psychiatric clinics, and private practitioners. All of these children have a major impairment in at least two areas of functioning (family, school, or peers). They need the 24-hour supervision of a hospital.

There are three general indications for admission to a short-term (3 weeks to 3 months) child psychiatry unit:

1. Protection of the child from himself or his parents
2. Severely aggressive behavior (towards others)
3. Intensive inpatient evaluation and treatment

Some children are brought to the hospital because of potentially harmful behavior such as running in front of cars, standing on a window ledge, wandering, self-abusive behavior, and taking pills. Even though the risk of suicide is small in children younger than preadolescence, the presence of such symptoms indicates either severe psychopathology and/or lack of parental supervision. A period of inpatient evaluation can clarify the nature of the problem and help decide a future course. Some children presenting with similar symptoms arouse suspicion of potential abuse from parents. Treatment in a psychiatric unit is a nonpunitive intervention that allows for the establishment of rapport with the child and parents while the child is in a protective setting. As a result of the evaluation, an appropriate long-term plan can be implemented.

The second major indication for hospitalization is severe aggressive behavior. Most of the children referred for hospitalization have some kind of severe behavioral disturbance that cannot be tolerated by the environment. The presenting symptoms and complaints include severe

17

temper tantrums at school or at home, aggression directed toward siblings or peers (e.g., threatening an infant sibling with a knife), inability of the parents and teachers to control the child, or excessive fighting. A period of 24-hour observation away from home can elucidate the etiology of the behavior disorder. The temporary separation between parent and child provides a "vacation" in order to restore a more harmonious equilibrium in the home.

The phrase "the child requires inpatient evaluation and treatment" is a catchall that is frequently used by referral sources. It can mean anything from "he's driving everybody up the wall, take him off our hands" to a carefully thought-out recommendation for 24-hour observation and treatment. A child may require hospitalization for several reasons. Outpatient treatment has either been unsuccessful, untenable, or the parents may not have been able to cooperate. This may occur for a variety of reasons: realistic shortage and limitations of once or twice weekly psychotherapy, family psychopathology that prevents cooperation with appointments and plans, or escalation of symptoms which cannot be understood and treated as an outpatient. At times, especially when a child is referred from another agency, it is difficult to assess whether failure of outpatient treatment has been due to the child's or family's psychopathology, mismatch of patient and therapist, or even the technical mishandling of a severely difficult case. In all of these situations 24-hour observation can pinpoint the child's and family's strengths and pathology.

It is crucial to assess the function of the child's symptoms within the family structure and balance. Not only the severity of the symptoms but the environment's response to the symptoms determine whether an inpatient evaluation is needed. Young children in particular present difficult problems because one is apt not to want to separate the child from his or her family. There are times, however, it is necessary to do this in order to curtail the continued trauma inflicted by an inadequate family which cannot contain the child.

A period of hospitalization can provide a detailed analysis of the child's general functioning, strengths, and deficits. The child is observed in relation to his or her peers, teachers, therapist, and other adults. Usually the child will reenact his or her conflicts with the staff and children on the ward. An in-depth understanding of the problem allows for therapeutic interventions by the various staff. At the same time this understanding is communicated to the family. The staff assesses the child's and family's response to treatment in order to decide whether outpatient, day, or residential treatment is the long-term treatment of choice.

For example, a 5½-year-old boy was referred by a social agency because of severe aggressive behavior, including attempts to harm a younger half brother. He had been placed in a foster home because his mother and stepfather could not handle his aggressiveness and were potentially, if not already, abusive toward him. Hospitalization was sought when the child's symptoms recurred in the foster home. Out-patient treatment (mostly medication) was not successful. It seemed clear that the degree of symptomatology plus the fragility of the home situation required intensive treatment. M. wanted to go back home. Daily home visits by the staff plus daily psychotherapy could have been an alternative to hospitalization. Since this was not possible for either Mount Sinai or the referring agency to accomplish, M. was hospitalized. Both M. and the parents became involved in intensive treatment. During the hospitalization, the parents were helped to understand M.'s sense of displacement, to begin to empathize with him, and to find methods other than hitting to help control him. The family and M. responded to the therapeutic interventions. After the 3-month hospitalization, M. returned home to continue outpatient family treatment with the same therapist.

On the other hand, J., another 5½-year-old boy, was admitted because of severe behavioral problems in a foster home. He had already been in a series of foster homes and his family was chaotic, inconsistent, and abusive in the past. His mother was unable to keep her appointment for parent-child activities. Since the family insisted that J. return home, the referral agency, with the hospital's aid, went to family court whereby J. was remanded for long-term residential treatment.

The intake process at the Mount Sinai Medical Center is planned and conducted with a view towards establishing a treatment alliance with the entire family. At the intake meeting a group of staff members from various disciplines review written material from the referring source. The family and child are interviewed jointly and separately in the outpatient department and then escorted to the unit where they are introduced to other staff members and shown the ward. A conference is conducted by the psychiatrist in charge of the unit, during which time a symptom and mental status checklist is completed. A preliminary diagnostic picture, specific problem areas, and tentative plans are formulated. If the child is not to be admitted to the unit the family is offered alternative treatment plans and assisted in following them up.

If the child is to be admitted to the unit, the staff members who are involved in the intake process usually retain primary responsibility for the treatment of the child and his or her family. At times, the child or the family is seen by the primary therapist between the screening appointment and the time of admission as part of a preparatory phase. This procedure is especially helpful in those situations in which symbiotic attachments between the parent and child may lead to undue anxiety in the parent and/or child upon separation. If a working alliance is not established with the parent prior to hospitalization, the ambivalence about hospitalization plus the anxiety generated by the separation may be so strong as to lead the parent to withdraw the child from the hospital setting.

Several problems arise during the intake procedure. The most crucial one involves the length of stay for children covered by Blue Cross. These children can only be hospitalized for 3 weeks and occasionally for 30 days. During this time a diagnostic profile can be formulated while the child and family are offered a temporary respite from a turmoil-filled situation. It is a great hardship, however, for the staff, families and especially for the children to be discharged right at the point where they have become adjusted to the unit and the staff has begun to understand them and their families. In a position statement on national health insurance, the American Academy of Child Psychiatry (1977, p. 6), recognized the problem of brief hospitalization. "It is important to emphasize here that duration of inpatient treatment for *children* is of a different magnitude from inpatient treatment of adults." Under present circumstances, the staff has to be aware that a very brief period of hospitalization can have only very limited goals.

A second problematic area involves children who are admitted on an emergency basis. Such children demonstrate some kind of destructive behavior (to self or others) that is acutely unmanageable to the care-takers in the child's environment. If the children do in fact enter the hospital on an emergency basis neither they nor their families can participate in the intake process. This has shown itself to be problematical.

If the child is admitted the same day he is brought into the emergency room, there is no time for the child or the family to come to terms with hospitalization. The crisis that required emergency attention often subsides quickly and the parent insists on a premature discharge without adequate posthospital planning. Most so-called emergencies with children respond to parental support and guidance. If at all possible, it is preferable for the child and parent to be able to participate in the intake procedure.

A final frequent problem has to do with children with severe behavior problems who have parents who have essentially abandoned them, or have been placed in foster homes or group homes. Wardle (1974) under the English system, suggested that such children should not be admitted to an inpatient hospital unless a home can be found prior to hospitalization. Then the goal of the hospitalization becomes one of helping the child enter the new family. This is not possible under our social structure. If such a system were to be established, the child would have to be able to stay in the hospital as long as necessary, not just 3 months. However, such children may profit from a 3-month hospitalization. During this time a major goal is to decide whether the child's behavior can be modified so that he would benefit from a foster home or whether long-term residential treatment is a better alternative. A regrettable consequence of the treatment of these children from extremely pathogenic unstable environments is that they become deeply attached to the hospital staff and therefore have difficulties in leaving. From intake onward, the staff must be aware of this in order to help the child recognize the temporary duration of his friendships in the hospital and to help him or her work through his or her affective distortions of the experience.

To summarize, the need for short-term psychiatric hospitalization for children usually arises out of a disequilibrium in a child's environment that results in making the child's symptoms unmanageable. The period of hospitalization allows for an in-depth understanding of the child's and family's strengths and deficits, therapeutic interventions to the child and family based on this understanding, and long-term planning based on the outcome of the inpatient evaluation.

REFERENCES

American Academy of Child Psychiatry (1977). *Position Statement on National Health Insurance*. Washington; D.C.

Sackin, H.D., and Meyer, A.D. (1976). Inpatient care for disturbed children: criteria for admission. Paper presented at American Academy of Child Psychiatry Annual Meeting. Toronto.

Silver, L.B., ed. (1976). *Professional Standards Review Organizations: A Handbook for Child Psychiatrists*. Washington, D.C.: American Academy of Child Psychiatry.

Wardle, C.J. (1974). Residential care of children with conduct disorders. In *The Residential Psychiatric Treatment of Children*. P. Barker, ed. New York: Halstead Press, pp. 48-104.

Chapter 4

THE ROLE OF THE CHILD PSYCHIATRIST AND THE CHILD PSYCHIATRY TRAINEE

Leon Hoffman
Paul Kennedy
Ronald Rawitt

The organization of the Child Psychiatry Inpatient Unit reflects its dual nature. On the one hand it provides service to severely disturbed children and their families based on the theoretical and practical principles detailed in this book. On the other hand, it provides education and training for child psychiatry fellows, for other students, and for regular staff members. There is an ongoing effort to conduct clinical research. A *medical model* is followed in that the unit is organized to facilitate *assessment* of the child and family, *diagnosis* (in a broad sense), and implementation of a *treatment plan*. The organization provides for the integration between the service, that is, the treatment, the teaching, and the training.

The staff of the unit consists of physicians (child psychiatrists, child psychiatry fellows, psychiatric residents, and pediatrician), psychiatric nurses, occupational and activity therapists, psychiatric social workers, special education teachers, and psychologists (Table 1). To facilitate working together and implementing a unified treatment plan, the unit personnel is divided into two teams. A child is assigned to a team, and within the team specified staff members take primary responsibility for the evaluation and treatment of that child ("miniteam").

The fellows or residents are usually the primary therapists (see Chap. 7). Since the focus is family-centered the cases are not "split." The primary therapist treats both the child and the family. The social workers provide consultation and supervision for the fellows, residents and other staff members of the work done with families. Some children are treated by social workers as the primary therapist. For them, the fellow or resident assumes medical responsibility including obtaining a detailed developmental and pediatric history.

Each child is assigned to a primary nurse (see Chap. 12), to a variety of structured and unstructured groups (see Chap. 9), and one of two small classes (see Chap. 11). The doctor, nurse, social worker, and therapeutic activities worker who function as a miniteam consult regularly for ongoing treatment planning. There is a coordinator (a senior clinical nurse) whose function is to ensure that the various conferences occur regularly and that the staff implement appropriate diagnostic and treatment plans.

It is self-evident that an active milieu which focuses on diagnosis, treatment, and teaching requires many meetings in order to *integrate*

TABLE 1

Staff Patterns of Child Psychiatry Unit

Administrative Staff (see Figure 1)

Attending Staff
   3 voluntary child psychiatry supervisors
   1 liaison pediatrician (voluntary staff)

Psychology
   3 part-time psychologists

School
   2 Board of Education teachers

Team A		Team B
Coordinator		Coordinator
Child Psychiatry Fellows/Residents:		
	2	2
Professional Nurses:		
Day Shift	4	3
Evening Shift	1	1
Midnight Shift	]1[	
Nursing Assistants:		
Day Shift	1	2
Evening Shift	1	1
Midnight Shift	]2[	
Therapeutic Activities:		
	1	1
Social Service:		
	2 (part-time)	2 (part-time)

Day Treatment Program

   Coordinator – Professional Nurse, Occupational Therapist,
      Board of Education Teacher; and
      Professional Nurse

the mass of data that is available and to implement successful treatment plans. All meetings focus on diagnosis, management, and therapy as well as teaching improved diagnostic and therapeutic skills.

Teaching occurs within the context of the evaluation and treatment process.

The senior staff can demonstrate a variety of techniques and focus discussions on appropriate topics. Two examples suffice: In the screening interview, one can demonstrate a way of dealing therapeutically with parental guilt over hospitalizing a child. During rounds, in a discussion of a negativistic child who doesn't pay attention to instructions, one can make all staff aware of possible auditory receptive problems as the cause of the child's "not listening." In this way, a rational treatment technique can be implemented by the staff and subsequently communicated to the parents.

An important tool in the education of staff is the use of videotaping.
All parents are asked to sign a permission form to allow videotaping of
themselves and their child. Very few parents refuse to do so. Groups,
families, and individual children are thus videotaped and techniques
reviewed with various staff members. The video may be conducted by
the particular therapist or by a senior staff such as the psychiatrist
in charge or the supervising social worker. For example, during a
monthly family conference, family interviewing techniques are demonstrated via a "live" family or a videotape.

One morning a week, two intake meetings are conducted. A
representative from each discipline is involved in a group interview of
the child and the family. The initial evaluation focuses on the child's
symptomatology, precipitants of current problems, and the family's
strengths and deficits in order to determine indications and goals of
hospitalization (see Appendix 1). The family, including the child, is
shown the unit and the case is discussed with the psychiatrist in
charge of the unit. Nearly always a decision can be made as to whether
hospitalization would be useful. Occasionally, more data is required
and follow-up appointments are arranged prior to making a decision
about hospitalization. If hospitalization is not advisable, appropriate
alternative recommendations are made.

Case conferences (rounds) are conducted three times a week. Each
child is discussed every other week except for the very brief admissions,
which are discussed weekly. The miniteams meet weekly in order to
follow up and implement plans which have been discussed at rounds.
At a weekly pediatric liaison meeting, general pediatric problems and
developmental issues are discussed with the attending pediatrician (see
Chap. 5). A weekly teachers' meeting allows for the integration of the
child's school program with the general treatment plan. In addition, a
weekly meeting is held during which time the group therapies and
general milieu treatments are discussed.

Charting follows the problem-oriented medical record format. At
the intake conference, problems are listed according to mental status
items (Appendix 2). Tentative treatment plans for the various problems
are formulated.

When the child is admitted to the hospital, a complete psychiatric
history is obtained by the primary therapist in conjunction with the
primary nurse. This includes basic identification and family data,
chief complaint, history of the present illness, past history, pediatric
history, developmental history (including play, activities, and interests),
family history and mental status (Appendix 3). If the primary therapist
is a nonphysician, the physician obtains the pediatric and developmental
history. A complete physical examination, including a special neurological
examination for motor "soft signs" is completed. Initial blood examina-
tions include complete blood counts, SMA-12, VDRL, and sickle cell
preparation for non-Caucasians. A urine analysis, tine test, and
throat culture (to prevent streptococcal group-A epidemics) are administered.

The problem list is updated at the time of admission, the indications
and goals of hospitalization are spelled out, and a plan is formulated.
All of this is detailed in the chart and updated biweekly treatment
plan (Appendix 4).

During the course of hospitalization, a psychological, sensori-motor
and developmental profile are obtained. Speech and hearing and neurological consultations are frequently requested. A formal diagnosis is
arrived at and a psychodynamic formulation postulated (Appendixes 5
and 6).

The primary therapist enters notes in the chart three times a week.
Other staff make entries as often as indicated. The notes include the
course of the child's and family problems, the child's behavior, interactions
with other children and staff, activities, school performance, and ongoing
result of the evaluations and consultations. The results of conferences
and supervisory sessions are recorded in the chart. The continued need
for hospitalization is thus documented.

Posthospital plans need to be considered from the beginning of the
hospitalization. Referral agencies and, when appropriate, the Bureau of
Child Welfare are invited to participate in the treatment and planning
discussions. The usual alternative plans include outpatient treatment by
the same therapist with or without special school placement, outpatient
treatment at another facility, day treatment at Mount Sinai or elsewhere,
group home or foster home, or residential treatment. The decision evolves
from the many staff discussions held on each child. A summary of the
course of evaluation is then sent to the appropriate agency.

THE CHILD PSYCHIATRIST

The experienced child psychiatrist is the person best equipped to
coordinate the program of a dynamic and developmentally oriented child
psychiatry unit (Berlin, 1978). In most residential treatment centers and
social agencies the psychiatrist is a consultant but not the coordinator.
Within the organizational schema of the Child Psychiatry Inpatient Unit
at Mount Sinai Medical Center the role and function of the psychiatrist in
charge is crucial. He or she is a role model for the child psychiatry
fellows and residents and other staff members. In this way, this person
coordinates the treatment, teaching, and research activities of the unit.

As is true in any organization the style of leadership will of course
affect the style and tone of the organizational structure. A balance needs
to be struck between directiveness and openness. The psychiatrist needs
to lead by consensus considering the various and, at times, diverse
opinions. At the same time he or she has to provide direction and an
overall frame of reference. The organization and structure of the unit
is dynamic and not static. The psychiatrist in charge needs to be flexible
in order to be able to implement necessary adaptations in the program.
In fact, there are constant adaptations and improvements. On the other
hand, the psychiatrist in charge needs to respond to contagious group
anxiety and "pseudo problems requiring change" not by implementing the
requested change but by supportive intervention with the staff, discouraging
emotional discussions of interpersonal staff issues, and redirection of
staff energies (Gruber, 1977).

On a milieu the different staff members view the child from a variety
of perspectives. Intrastaff conflicts may arise out of a competitiveness
as to whose point of view is most valid. A common example prevalent in
any child care institution involves the different perspective between the
psychotherapist and the day-to-day worker. The child often interacts
quite differently with the different staff. A major teaching goal is to help
the staff utilize the *apparently* contradictory observations in implementing
a unified treatment plan. In the dynamic of a milieu, the staff needs to
understand that in the decision-making process all points of view are
considered. Whenever a consensus cannot be reached, however, someone
needs to make a final decision.

In the organizational structure of the general hospital each discipline
is administratively responsible to its own hierarchy (Fig. 1). For example,
the supervising social worker is directly responsible to the hierarchy of
the social service department. In the actual day-to-day treatment of the

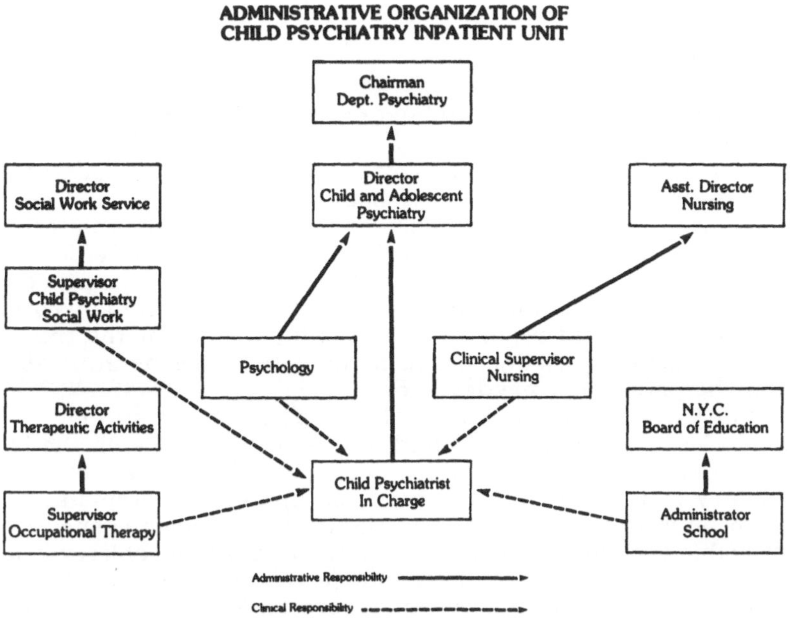

ADMINISTRATIVE ORGANIZATION OF
CHILD PSYCHIATRY INPATIENT UNIT

Fig. 1.

children and in the general area of program planning and development
the child psychiatrist provides leadership for the various disciplines.
To this end, a weekly supervisory meeting is held in order to integrate
the thinking of the various disciplines and resolve interdisciplinary conflicts. The psychiatrist in charge of the unit conducts the meeting. The
supervisory social worker, the nursing clinical supervisor, the supervising
occupational therapist, the supervising child psychologist, the school
administrator, and the director of the Division of Child Psychiatry attend
this meeting. General program plans and policies are discussed at this
meeting. The function of the day treatment program is supervised at
this meeting and an attempt is made to coordinate the inpatient and day
patient treatment with the rest of the outpatient department.

It is crucial for the psychiatrist in charge of the unit to have direct
contact with all staff on the unit. On a unit with a large number of staff,
general staff meetings are usually not productive because effective work
cannot be accomplished with this large number of people. Furthermore,
if conflicting issues are discussed, unresolvable feelings may be generated
which worsen rather than help intrastaff conflicts. Therefore, small
staff meetings are conducted within the various disciplines. The psychiatrist in charge meets with the various staff on a regular and ad hoc
basis and provides input to the various disciplines.

In addition to the psychiatrist in charge of the unit, three experienced
child psychiatrists provide supervision for the child psychiatry fellows
and residents. These child psychiatrists each attend one of the rounds
and provide supervision to the fellows and residents for individual psychotherapy. Since the psychiatrists attend the rounds, they are able to
help the trainee integrate the individual's psychotherapy with the general
milieu plan. A monthly meeting is conducted during which time the
supervising child psychiatrists meet with the supervising social worker,
the psychiatrist in charge of the unit, and the director of child psychiatry
in order to integrate the teaching and supervising functions and provide

for ways in which to help the fellows and residents if problems arise.

THE CHILD PSYCHIATRY TRAINEE*

The inpatient unit provides a unique setting for the child psychiatry trainee to learn about disturbed latency children. Many of the children have serious delays or deviations in their development. The fellow is able to gain special insights into the 24-hour-a-day experience of his or her child patients. The total experience of the child can be monitored: his peer and adult relationships, school functioning, play activities, and daily life chores. This is in contrast to the trainee's experience in the outpatient department, where information about the child is colored by the biases of the parent reporter. On the inpatient unit the trainee can see the immediate correlation between the data he learns in psychotherapy sessions and the patient's everyday life.

On the inpatient unit the child psychiatry fellow has a special opportunity to learn techniques of child psychotherapy. He or she is provided with extensive experience in working with other members of an interdisciplinary team, including teachers, occupational therapists, psychologists, social workers, nurses, and members of various agencies. This is invaluable training for his future work in child psychiatry. He or she learns to integrate data and coordinate treatment plans. The child fellow can learn practical behavioral maneuvers for dealing with disturbed children in everyday situations. He or she learns to appreciate the value of timely and appropriate limit-setting. The fellow can then transmit this information to the parents. Medications can be titrated to suit the individual child's needs and thereby increase the training fellow's skills as a psycho-pharmacologist.

The experience on the inpatient unit sharpens the fellow's skills as a teacher. He or she teaches the child new ways of coping and teaches the other staff the meaning of the child's behavior as understood via the uniqueness of a psychotherapeutic relationship. The structure of the unit allows for quick feedback about the success or failure of specific interventions be they behavioral, psychodynamic, pharmacologic, or family oriented, thus teaching the fellow about the efficacy of his or her therapeutic interventions.

Through his or her participation in the milieu, the trainee can learn about children's lives in a special way. He or she observes and participates in children's group activities, both formal and informal, in play, and in talking situations. The fellow experiences him- or herself as a parental surrogate as well as a therapist in these groups, gaining a better understanding of the child's family life and the child's feelings about his family situation. The fellow can better empathize with the parents because he shares a parental role on the inpatient unit.

In working on an inpatient child psychiatry unit one not only has the opportunity to work with the "parent," but also with the family. The fellow needs to have contact with the family. Information is gathered about the family through the expression of their concern about their hospitalized child. This allows for special therapeutic interventions with both the family and child. Sometimes a change in symptoms occurs when the child is admitted to the inpatient unit and separated from his family, however, the child's symptoms can change as he adjusts to living in the hospital "family." Separating the child from his family starts the process of "teasing out" environmental from innate factors. The fellow learns how to help parents help their child.

---

*The material in this section was contributed by Paul Kennedy and Ronald Rawitt.

The contributions of environmental and innate factors to the child's psychopathology is aided by the various testing procedures in addition to round-the-clock observation. The tests include psychological, neurological, speech and hearing, and perceptual-motor testing.

The experience on the child inpatient unit allows the child fellow to be totally involved in the daily lives of children and yet maintain a necessary clinical perspective. This total approach enhances the sophistication, breadth, and depth of his clinical skills.

During the second year of the child fellowship, the fellow functions as the consultant to the day treatment program under the supervision of the psychiatrist in charge. In contrast to the first-year experience, the fellow learns during this second year how to digest and integrate data from other mental health professionals and communicate meaningful suggestions to them. This role is an important one of the child psychiatrist in many agencies. On the one hand, one cannot retreat to the stance that the therapist does not have enough data for the consultant to evaluate. On the other hand, one cannot make suggestions based on pat hypothetical formulations.

The child psychiatric fellow thus learns from intensive involvement on the inpatient unit and from consultative involvement in the day treatment program.

REFERENCES

Berlin, I.N. (1978). Developmental issues in the psychiatric hospitalization of children. *Am. J. Psychiatry 135:* 1044-1048.

Gruber, L.N. (1977). An organizational distress syndrome: Diagnosis and treatment. *Hosp. Commun. Psychiatry 28:* 517-521.

Chapter 5

PEDIATRIC LIAISON

Robert M. Berk

"What is specific to psychiatry as a medical discipline is its responsibility for the biologic as well as the psychologic aspects of behavior;
what is specific to child psychiatry is its concern for an organism whose
body, brain and mind interact profoundly with the process of development."
This statement by Leon Eisenberg (1965) indicates clearly the importance
of the medical foundations upon which the child psychiatrist must construct
the evaluation of his or her patient.

In the case of children, these medical foundations are derived from
pediatrics, and one would presume that close ties between the two
disciplines, child psychiatry and pediatrics, would be taken for granted.
However, this has not been the general situation. A review of the history
of child psychiatry reveals a very interesting pattern of evolution in its
interaction with pediatrics.

The initial inpatient psychiatric services for children in the United
States were established to care for children who suffered from post-
encephalitic behavior disorders following an epidemic of encephalitis
lethargica at the end of World War I (American Psychiatric Association,
1957). In the ensuing years a gradual change was effected in the function
of child care institutions because of the observations of the developmental
distortion of personality in children raised in institutional settings.
From simply providing custodial care, these homes began to offer psychiatric
help for children with emotional problems. This was the first step in the
evolution of several of the functioning child care institutions into residential
psychiatric treatment centers.

Descriptions of these therapeutic settings present the interdisciplinary
team of psychiatry, psychology, nursing, education, and social work.
Apparently, pediatrics was not considered a part of inpatient psychiatric
therapy. Even some recent publications do not include the pediatrician
as a work partner (Barker, 1974; Bettleheim, 1950; Blau and Slaff, 1964;
Copus and Walker, 1972; Evangelakis, 1974; Stratas and Schmidt, 1960;
Treffert, 1969). A descriptive study of the *major* existing residential
centers for emotionally disturbed children (Reid and Hagar, 1952),
presented a very disturbing picture. Most of the centers did not have a
pediatrician on staff. Most used locally available medical facilities for
acute and chronic care of their patients. Of the 12 institutions described,
only three were regularly staffed with some sort of pediatric service and
only one, the Emma Pendleton Bradley Home in Providence, Rhode Island,

29

whose director was a pediatrician, was regularly staffed by pediatric
residents as well as child psychiatry trainees.

However, this evident lack of pediatric presence in inpatient child
care was noted in the Conference on Training in Child Psychiatry (1963).
There it was emphasized that "child psychiatry in all its aspects is most
closely associated with medicine, general psychiatry, and other medical
specialties, notably pediatrics" (sic). The preoccupation of those concerned
with child welfare with the emotional problems of the child causes them
to overlook the importance of the physical body in the lives of the children
(Whittaker and Treischman, 1972). "We have overlooked physical health
or illness as part of the normal development or as the continuation of
previous attempts to cope with stress. Thus, in residential treatment
instead of unifying psyche and soma and treating the child as a whole,
we have continually kept these two apart, as if the twain never shall meet."
Bettleheim (1950) and Anna Freud (1970), among others, emphasize the
importance of interaction between psyche and soma. Thus, in the general
care and treatment of children, no matter what their problem, a total
approach through all modalities is required in order to provide each child
with the optimum care to which he or she is entitled.

Looking back, one observes that "up to approximately 1930, psychiatry
was not integrated with the rest of medicine, and pediatrics saw in medical
psychology nothing that it might incorporate into itself except intelligence
testing. Pediatricians were still teaching parents the tenets of behaviorism,
although the parents themselves were beginning to question, and even
resist advice about child care which was rigid, artificial, mechanical and
fitted to animal experimentation in the conditioning experiment rather
than to a home and parent-child relationship" (Senn, 1946).

In 1946, the teaching program at New York Hospital for pediatric
psychiatry attempted to alter the then-current approach. Attempts were
made to include the following basic topics in the program: (1) recognition
of the mental (emotional, social, and intellectual) growth and behavior of
infants from birth to maturity with consideration of heredity, somatic,
psychological, interpersonal, and cultural forces which take place in the
development of each person from conception onward; (2) understanding
the psychological implication of childbearing and rearing, education,
and child care in health and sickness, especially in terms of parent-child
relationships but including other interpersonal relationships of the parent
and child; (3) observing the psychological concomitants of physical illness
and the psychological role of the physician and nurse in parental guidance
and in medical treatment of sick children and adolescents; and (4) an
awareness of deviant personality structure and psychopathology, especially
in psychosomatic relationships, with emphasis on the genesis, prevention
and treatment of emotional difficulties and so-called behavior problems of
all age groups from birth to adolescence. It is quite obvious that basic
fundamentals of pediatric knowledge are mandatory to successful training.

In the Conference on Training in Child Psychiatry (1963) a number of
reasons were outlined for the uniqueness of child psychiatry as a discipline.
The child psychiatrist requires a continual awareness of the importance
of physical and emotional growth and maturation to a child's functioning
and the constant relevance of developmental phase to the child's thinking,
feeling, and behaving. There must also be the knowledge that there are
multiple physical, intellectual, and emotional lines of development in the
growing child and that development in these areas may not proceed at
equal rates. *A special understanding of how children normally develop
is essential to prognosis and treatment.* There must also be a knowledge
of the physical and psychological aspects of normal and pathological develop-

ment and of the interaction of the multiple forces of health and disease. As a physician, the child psychiatrist should be able to perceive both physical and emotional factors as they interact in the etiology and sequelae of illness. He or she must also have the capacity to collaborate with other medical and nonmedical professional disciplines, pediatricians and other physicians, psychiatric social workers, clinical psychologists, and nurses and teachers in comprehensive diagnosis and treatment of children. There must be an *understanding that the goal of the child psychiatrist is not just the immediate relief of clinical symptoms but more fundamentally, the removal of roadblocks to the child's continual growth, enabling him to progress securely through succeeding developmental stages.* The ultimate goal is prevention of illness. This may be accomplished by various means, for example, parent education, early detection and treatment of disease and research.

As a physician, the child psychiatrist is concerned with the medical history and the diagnosis of physical disease as part of his or her final medical responsibility for total diagnosis and treatment. The fact that the normally immature patient is rapidly growing and developing, both physically and psychobiologically, poses special problems in differential diagnosis for the child psychiatrist. As a diagnostician, he or she must continually evaluate the child's ever-changing thinking, feelings, and behavior in the light of expected patterns for his or her stage of development.

An important clinical function is the child psychiatrist's appraisal of the child's physical status, and his ultimate responsibility for the medical history, the physical examination, and any special diagnostic studies. The child psychiatrist should have a thorough knowledge of physical diagnosis in children and at least normal competency in performing the physical examination. *Physical examination including neurological evaluation during the initial diagnostic period* can yield helpful information, not only about the child's physical status, but also about his or her emotional response to the situation and his or her various body parts.

In most instances, referral to a competent pediatrician is routine practice for the average child psychiatrist. The decision as to the necessity of such a referral must be based on careful mature clinical judgement. The *pediatrician may then contribute his skills to the comprehensive diagnosis and, through ongoing physical care, to the total treatment of the patient.*

The present inpatient unit for child psychiatry at Mount Sinai Medical Center has been in existence for over 15 years. This author has been actively affiliated with that service during those years. It is of interest to note that an early article describing the service (Blau and Slaff, 1964) does not mention pediatric liaison but does refer to the importance of the availability of pediatric consultation. However, over the years the role of the pediatrician has evolved into one which is an integral part of the unit. The skills of the pediatrician are utilized by many members of the therapeutic team, that is, child psychiatrists, both those in training and supervisory personnel, the nursing staff, and the social workers.

The presence of a psychiatric service for children distinct from the pediatric service in the hospital provides numerous advantages both to staff and children. The placement of psychiatric patients on a regular pediatric ward is not suitable for seriously disturbed, psychotic, homicidal, suicidal, or very aggressive patients (American Academy Pediatrics, 1971). Their needs differ from children in general pediatrics. Severely physically ill children with psychiatric problems are best handled, at least temporarily, on the pediatric service. Once the acute medical problem has been controlled, these children can then be admitted to the psychiatric service where continuing pediatric care is provided, supervised by the liaison pediatrician.

The role of the pediatrician on the unit is twofold; first as an instructor, providing much needed information to the psychiatric fellow, and second as a medical supervisor. Pediatrics provides exposure to the developmental viewpoint and experience in assessing normality and its variations. It increases competence in evaluating the significance of biological factors in psychological development and its aberration. It provides experience with physical illness, especially chronic illness, and its impact on personality development. It prepares the child psychiatry fellow to assume medical responsibility toward the child and family.

Continuous exposure to pediatrics during the course of training in child psychiatry is essential, particularly within the framework of well-baby care and the developmental examination (Conference on Training in Child Psychiatry, 1963). Pediatric instruction should contribute to adequacy in differential diagnosis by providing a knowledge of systemic disorders and brain syndromes.

Appreciation that the future is likely to bring increasing knowledge of biological and physical factors in childhood mental illness places an additional emphasis on the value of pediatric training and the necessity for the fellow of keeping abreast of new developments and their relevance for clinical practice.

The ideal training center for child psychiatry should be actively involved in the pediatric service of a general hospital or be part of a children's hospital (Conference on Training in Child Psychiatry, 1963). Pediatricians have the unique opportunity to observe individual differences in behavior patterns; varying child-rearing practices and their consequences; the emergence of curiosity, learning patterns, coping behavior, and personality; and the capacities of children and families to master adversity. These observations, made continually in the daily work of pediatrics, can prove invaluable to the accruing knowledge of the child psychiatry fellow (Richmond, 1967).

Physical care and continuing health supervision provided in any inpatient center for children is determined in large part by the auspices under which the institution operates (American Psychiatric Association, 1957). Some centers depend on the medical services of the physician, pediatric or otherwise, in the community. Others use personnel from an affiliated hospital. However, continuous service by one pediatric consultant is preferable. It is desirable for the pediatrician to be a member of the staff on a full-time or part-time basis, according to the size of the center.

The function of the pediatric liaison is to provide medical supervision of the child's health and to supervise the treatment of intercurrent infection and illness. As part of the admission evaluation of each patient, information is obtained regarding general development and previous pediatric medical history. Every effort is made to obtain the immunization records on each child. If such information is not available, or if the patients are not completely immunized, we attempt to protect all patients with up-to-date tetanus and polio immunizations. Measles, mumps, and rubella immunization status is determined as well, and protection is provided where necessary. Tine tuberculin testing is performed as is a complete blood count, urinalysis, sickle cell evaluation, serology, and SMA-12. This information provides a baseline with which future comparisons can be made as these children are followed. Side effects of psychotropic drugs, which may alter laboratory findings, can be readily observed with such a baseline comparison.

The general nutritional state of each child is noted and appropriate dietary management is provided. Should special measures be required, the services of the dietary department of the hospital are utilized.

Individual diets for obese children, the anorectic, allergic or diabetic child, or any other child requiring special management, is always available.

Following the initial workup of each child, attempts are made to provide optimal care of the child's physical health and integrate such care with psychiatric management. The presence of any correctable physical anomalies must be evaluated and treated using any of the varied specialized services that are part of the hospital. In addition, the psychiatric staff is provided with data on the child's biological endowment and capacity for use in planning the total treatment program. The liaison pediatrician assists in training clinical and child care personnel so that all staff members may have a better understanding of the physical concomitants of psychological disorders and their treatment.

In collaboration with the psychiatric staff, the pediatrician helps evaluate the complete physical examination of each child on admission. He helps supervise the health facilities and living and recreational facilities. Particular attention is paid to accident prevention and the prompt management of accidents, should they occur. There is particularly close continuing supervision and assistance in planning for children with special medical problems such as hearing or visual losses, rheumatic disease, orthopedic problems, and so on. The management of infectious disease and the care of children with allergies in collaboration with the psychiatric staff is most important. Decisions need to be made concerning isolation procedures, medication, and the routes of administration as well as the meaning to the patient and the timing of surgical and other procedures. Whether or not a physically sick child should remain on the unit or be transferred to the general pediatric service is carefully evaluated by both the psychiatrist and pediatrician.

In order to adequately treat children with a variety of problems, emphasis must be placed on the concept of the whole patient. One cannot compartmentalize problems into divisible sections. For example, asthma is multidetermined. It can be provoked in susceptible patients by a wide variety of different stresses, physical irritants, upper respiratory infections, allergies, or emotional stress. Bronchospasms may not occur unless more than one stress is operating, that is, infection plus emotion, and so on (Vaughn and McKay, 1975).

One must review all the etiologic factors in assessing psychosomatic disorders. One must remember that no one specific emotional problem is the cause of bronchospasm. Emotional problems may vary and the response may be the same. There is a nonspecificity of emotional stress, as opposed to the specificity of allergy, infection, and other physical conditions. It is most important for medical evaluation of the symptom pattern to be carefully processed to understand the nature of causative factors.

In order to understand parental attitudes towards symptoms and disease with psychosomatic disorders, an adequate history must be obtained. It is also important for the physician to relieve parental and patient anxiety regarding these conditions. In the treatment of such problems the pediatrician must be willing to work closely with the psychiatrist. He must accept the fact that alleviation of symptoms does not treat the underlying emotional factors. Therefore, a balance must be achieved. Symptomatic measures must not be misrepresented as cures. The integration of medical and psychiatric therapy is most important. There must be progressive liaison between the disciplines of pediatrics and child psychiatry so that each reinforces the contribution of the other (Pinkertin, 1965).

Pinkertin (Barket, 1974) indicates three main categories of illness that one is liable to encounter in which the interaction of medical and psychiatric problems occur. First, the somatopsychic disorders, such as neuroepilepsy, cystic fibrosis, diabetes mellitus, urogenital anomalies, orthopedic lesion, Hirschsprung's disease, and hyperthyroidism. In these, the lesion is primarily organic, but may give rise to disturbed behavior. This may occur in a direct fashion as with the chemical derangement and body response in hyperthyroidism. It may also occur due to patient acceptance or nonacceptance of the organic disease. The child's behavior may be affected by parental reaction to the disease. Psychological stress in childhood is often associated with physical illness or handicap present at birth or because of early onset. Sensitive pediatric handling can plan a preventive role in minimizing or eliminating destructive behavioral adaptation, that is, adjustment to serious orthopedic abnormalities, allergy, rheumatic fever, blindness, deafness, and so on. Psychological response to illness may sometimes intensify organic conditions, for example, diabetes — failure of the child to stay on a diet or medication.

The second category Pinkertin calls the pseudosomatic. In this group he includes enuresis, encopresis, recurrent abdominal pain, obesity, hysteria, tics, alopecia, anorexia, cardiac neuroses, hypochondriasis, and so on. Here parental attitude antedates the problem, ranging from overinvolvement to rejection. The child then reacts accordingly.

The third category encompasses the true psychosomatic disorders. These include asthma, eczema, abdominal migraine and cyclic vomiting, peptic ulcer, and ulcerative colitis. Here both organic and psychological factors are important. By observation one can determine the degree to which each operates. The importance of total evaluation, medical and psychiatric, cannot be overemphasized.

At Mount Sinai Medical Center, short-term hospitalization is the rule, ranging from 3 weeks to 3 months. As pointed out by Laybourne and Miller (1962) such periods can have both diagnostic and therapeutic implications for emotionally disturbed children. These authors hospitalized children with emotional problems in a general pediatric hospital for a period of several days to a few months to clarify difficult diagnostic questions and to help resolve emotional problems which otherwise might not be resolved on an outpatient basis. They observed that hospitalization of children in psychiatrically oriented children's hospitals will often bring about remission in symptomatology. This is particularly true in the psychosomatic disorders such as cyclic vomiting, ulcerative colitis, and bronchial asthma. The authors indicate the temporary nature of the improvement in symptoms and emphasize that one must deal with the underlying problems for a permanent solution. As to the question of separation, "short term separation of parent and child in selected cases can allow movement which might not occur under other circumstances. This is particularly true for preschool children suffering from acute emotional disturbance. These children often respond dramatically to a few days in the hospital." This proves true for both medical and psychiatric symptoms.

Another area other than the psychosomatic in which the pediatrician can be helpful is associated with genetic disease. For example, the behavioral picture of phenylketonuria may resemble certain features of other syndromes, including childhood schizophrenia. The disease may manifest itself in psychotic behavior, mental retardation, or seizures, as well as unusually light pigmentation and eczema, or may present itself in various combinations. Down's syndrome, Turner's syndrome, and Klinefelter's syndrome are other genetic disorders which may appear in the psychiatric setting. Chromosomal breaks due to ingestion of drugs may also affect offspring (Cohen, Hirschhorn, and Frosh, 1967) and their consideration must also be included in evaluation of the patient.

"The psychologically oriented pediatrician is in a position to function as a preventive psychiatrist. Since he observes behavior patterns in their formative stages, it is possible for him to encourage or discourage the development of particular trends. It is he who usually has the first opportunity to recognize the emergence of destructive patterns of behavior, such as morbid dependency, self-depreciation, or unhealthy expression of hostility" (Chess, 1969).

The child psychiatrist needs to keep his knowledge of pediatrics up to date. It is now recognized that organic difficulties may play a far greater role in the genesis of psychiatric disorders than was previously suspected, and the relationship between physical illness and disturbance in behavior is becoming more obvious. To understand fully the effect a particular physical illness may have on behavior requires a familiarity with pediatric disease syndromes. The child psychiatrist must be equally aware of the effect that past illness and treatment may have on the child's behavior. He must be alert to the signs of physical illness in children. He must be able to evaluate the fundamental facts in the pediatric picture.

Thus, the training of the child psychiatrist requires pediatric liaison and consultation experience. By doing so one hopes to "establish the basis for effective communication in the training years for both of these key disciplines responsible for the optimal development of our country's children" (Lourie, 1966).

REFERENCES

American Psychiatric Association (1957). *Psychiatric Inpatient Treatment of Children.* Baltimore: Lord Baltimore.

Barker, P. (1974). *The Residential Psychiatric Treatment of Children.* New York: Wiley.

Bettleheim, B. (1950). *Love is not Enough.* Glencoe, Ill.: The Free Press.

Blau, A., and Slaff, B. (1964). Child psychiatry division in a general hospital. *N.Y. State J. Med. 64:*1096-1100.

American Academy of Pediatrics (1971). *Care of Children in Hospital,* 2nd ed., Washington, D.C.

Chess, S. (1969). *An Introduction to Child Psychiatry.* New York: Grune & Stratton.

Cohen, M.M., Hirschhorn, K., and Frosh, W.A. (1967). In vivo and in vitro chromosomal damage induced by LSD-25. *N. Engl. J. Med. 277(20):*1043-1049.

Conference on Training in Child Psychiatry. Washington, D.C., January 10-15, 1963.

Copus, P.E., and Walker, W.L. (1972). The psychiatric ward in a children's hospital: A review of the first two years. *Br. J. Psychiatry 212:*323-326.

Eisenberg, L. (1967). The relationship between psychiatry and pediatrics: A disputatious view. *Pediatrics 39:*645-647.

Evangelakis, M. (1974). *A Manual for Residential and Day Treatment of Children.* Springfield, Ill.: Charles C Thomas.

Freud, A. (1970). The symptomatology of children. In *Psychoanalytic Study of the Child;* Vol. 25. New York: N.Y. Int. Univ. Press; pp. 19-41.

Jones, M. (1953). *The Therapeutic Community: A New Treatment Method in Psychiatry.* New York: Basic Books.

Laybourne, P.C., and Miller, H. (1962). Pediatric hospitalization of psychiatric patients: Diagnostic and therapeutic implication. *Am. J.*

*Orthopsychiatry 32:*596-603.

Lourie, R.S. (1966). Problems of diagnosis and treatment — Communication between pediatrician and psychiatrist. *Pediatrics 37:*1000-1004.

Pinkertin, P. (1965). The psychosomatic approach in child psychiatry. In *Modern Perspectives in Child Psychiatry*. J.G. Howells, ed. Edinburgh: Olver and Beryd, pp. 306-335.

Reid, J.H., and Hagar, H.R. (1952). *Residential Treatment of Emotionally Disturbed Children: A Descriptive Study*. New York: Child Welfare League of America.

Richmond, J.B. (1967). Child development: A basic science for pediatrics. *Pediatrics 39:*649-658.

Senn, M.J.E. (1946). Relationships of pediatrics and psychiatry. *Am. J. Dis. Child. 71:*537-549.

Stratas, N.E., and Schmidt, K.J. (1960). A children's unit in a state hospital. *Am. J. Psychiatry 117:*34-36.

Treffert, D.A. (1969). Child-adolescent unit in a psychiatric hospital. *Arch. Gen. Psychiatry 21:*745-752.

Vaughn, V.C., and McKay, R.J., eds. (1975). *Nelson Textbook of Pediatrics*, 10th ed. Philadelphia: Saunders.

Whittaker, J., and Treisschman, A., eds. (1972). *Children Away From Home: A Source Book in Residential Treatment*. Chicago: Aldrich.

Chapter 6

DEVELOPMENTAL AND DIAGNOSTIC ASSESSMENT

Robyn Abramson

Children who are hospitalized on a short-term psychiatric unit usually demonstrate diagnostic and therapeutic problems. Short-term hospitalization of the child serves the purpose of (1) evaluation and diagnosis, (2) short-term treatment and crisis intervention for the child and family, and (3) disposition planning. Evaluation and treatment occur simultaneously and both processes remain ongoing throughout the period of hospitalization.

During the initial phase the staff arrives at a treatment plan, based on the tentative diagnostic, developmental and psychodynamic assessment of the child and family formulated during the screening and admission procedures. It is particularly important that the diagnosis take into consideration the child's level of development, developmental arrests and strengths, as well as the child's capacity to engaged in and utilize a psychotherapeutic relationship. As hospitalization is short term, it becomes even more essential that an early developmental assessment be undertaken (Berlin, 1978). A careful developmental assessment, utilizing the data from the various aspects of the milieu, must arrive at an understanding of the child's ego-functioning and level of defensive organization, his capacity for and level of object relationships, the extent of superego development and lacunae, and the degree of regression and levels of fixation (A. Freud, 1965).

In order to effectively implement a rational diagnostic and therapeutic process the staff must be trained in developmental theory in an ongoing way. It is not enough to say, for example, that a child functions below his developmental level or that his ego functions are impaired. The staff must learn to identify behaviors that are age-appropriate as well as those that are not (Appendix 7). In this way a variety of ego functions are evaluated according to general developmental norms (Appendix 6).

There are functions such as sensory (perceptual), motor cognitive/ language, social (object relations), and morality (superego), that we have found to be of particular diagnostic and prognostic importance. Similar to Chritchley and Berlin (1979), we have found that it is crucial to evaluate the nature of the child's social relations.

From the first contact with the unit staff, the child reveals the quality of his object relations. For example, a child may separate too easily from his or her family or have a severe panic reaction upon separating. On the unit, he or she may be a loner, form indiscriminate attachments, cling to adults, and so on. If the child can establish a meaningful relationship with someone on the unit, that child would be more likely to do well postdischarge.

Other ego functions which are particularly crucial to evaluate include the child's ability to differentiate thought from action (reality testing), his mode of thinking and comprehension of cause and effect, as well as an evaluation of his play skills.

Most of the children hospitalized have suffered severe and early deprivation and trauma; for such children the central intrapsychic issues revolve around loss, separation, and fears of annihilation. They are terrified of their own aggression, as well as of threatened loss of control. Many already display significant regression, and many have never developed adequate internal controls. They have difficulty differentiating thought from action and comprehending cause and effect.

One 9-year-old child was hospitalized after a period of severe aggressive outbursts directed at his mother and younger sibling (a prototypical chief complaint). His rage reached the proportion of murderous impulses, with both the child and mother totally unable to handle the experience. These outbursts of rage resulted in part after a trial of outpatient psychotherapy in which the child had been allowed to discharge rage indiscriminately and no limits had been set. This patient's high level of intelligence and his good verbal capacity masked a more serious borderline syndrome. The primary difficulty was the child's inability to integrate aggressive and libidinal impulses and to control these outbursts. The focus of the therapy in conjunction with the milieu treatment during the initial phase of hospitalization became an effort at developing better ego control, and was geared to assisting the child in developing a more adequate defensive structure, improving reality testing, and improving his capacity for delay and frustration tolerance. This child's aggression was controlled in order for him to experience being controlled and then ultimately controlling himself. This external aid provided for the child in order to compensate for his developmental defect led to some improvement in the child's functioning, and ultimately it became possible to help him deal more effectively with his rage reaction.

In addition to the clinical assessment, standardized tests provide much valuable information. These tests offer the staff concrete data to enable them to refine their assessments and plan for treatment. They help identify specific components of disturbed behaviors which are integrated with the clinical evaluation in order to formulate a comprehensive treatment plan. Often, the results of standardized tests confirm clinical impressions but, whenever a discrepancy occurs, further formal and clinical evaluation is needed.

Standardized tests are performed within the context of a structured situation. This often influences the child's behavior and thus his or her performance on the test. A negative child, a paranoid child, or one who needs control over his environment may be resistant to the testing sessions. This kind of a response to a testing situation may be correlated to the child's response to a formal structure such as a classroom setting. On the other hand, many deprived children demonstrate their greatest potential in this kind of setting because they receive positive reinforcement from any one-to-one relationship, no matter how brief an encounter.

Generally, formal testing sessions are deferred until a week after admission. This delay allows the child time for an adjustment to the unit and thus maximizes his or her performance level. Unlike outpatients, hospitalized children require more frequent and shorter testing sessions because poor concentration and decreased attention span interferes with performance. Each child must be prepared for each testing session.

Group discussions and explanations about the testing often help diminish test anxiety.

One of the difficulties in evaluating the results of the standardized tests is the cultural variance among a low socioeconomic population. A bilingual upbringing or an impoverished setting may impair a child's performance on some of the intelligence subtests. A standard score may be invalid if the child did not understand the instructions or if veralizations are expected from a child who was raised primarily in a nonverbal environment. With such children, nonverbal tasks provide a closer approximation of their general intelligence than do verbal tasks. However, the lack of age-adequate verbal skills is a major impediment to the development of many of the children on the unit. Thus, the results of the psychological testing provide a clue as to which areas the child is deficient in, in order to provide remediation.

The psychologist administers a battery of tests geared to the age of the child. The standard battery consists of the

1. Bender-Gestalt test
2. Human figure drawings (two genders, and sometimes a drawing of "the worst concept")
3. Intelligence test
   (a) WISC or WISC-R
   (b) WPPSI and/or Merril-Palmer (for younger children)
4. Rorschach
5. TAT, or Michigan Picture test, or CAT (depending on the age level)

The goal of the psychological evaluation is to achieve an understanding and diagnostic assessment of a child's intellectual and emotional functioning. Psychodynamics, intrapsychic conflicts, defenses, personality styles, and a degree of organicity are primary components extrapolated from this material. The projective tests sometimes show greater intellectual potential in the child (such as his or her level of organization or imagination) than formal intellectual tests.

Psychological tests offer information not readily observable in the clinical setting. For example, latent strengths and weaknesses are often revealed. A child may appear clinically retarded but his or her performance on tests may show good intellectual functioning. On the other hand, it is valuable for the clinicians to be aware of psychopathology which may not be evident clinically.

In interpreting the data from a psychological battery, the clinician looks for intercorrelations, patterns, and discrepancies in test scores. It is essential to utilize a total battery of tests, which evaluates all functions.

The psychological evaluation is an aid to the therapeutic team in order to help determine the best course of treatment for each child. The intelligence tests help influence academic placements. The other tests help identify a child's ego strengths, level of self-awareness, and motivation for change. The psychological battery may also help in the decision as to what may be the best form of psychotherapy: supportive, insight oriented, verbal, nonverbal, and so on.

The occupational therapist administers a battery of tests to assess perceptual skills and level of sensory integration. These areas are precursors of academic learning because they enable the child to "receive, filter, and organize sensory stimuli so as to make an adaptive response to the environment" (Ayres, 1973). A child with perceptual problems may misperceive the environment and respond with inappropriate behaviors such as hyperactivity, irritability, withdrawal, tactile defensiveness, spinning, and head banging. These aberrant behaviors are often the precipitants for referral to a psychiatric clinic or hospital. Clinicians must recognize and consider perceptual deficits as variables contributing to emotional disturbance, resulting in inappropriate behavior.

The *Southern California Test of Sensory Integration* (Ayres, 1973) is the primary battery for evaluating perceptual dysfunction. This battery evaluates subcortical functions within the visual/spatial, tactile/kinesthetic, vestibular, and motor domains.

Results from this battery provide a specialized neurophysiological diagnosis which delineates focal areas for treatment. The occupational therapist recommends appropriate interventions to teachers, parents, and clinicians in order to aid them in understanding, teaching, and managing effectively perceptually impaired children. Occupational therapy treatment focuses on the remediation of these perceptual problems through sensory stimulation and activities which facilitate an adaptive motor response (Ayres, 1973) to the environment in order to help the child compensate for his or her deficit.

The occupational therapist also administers formal developmental evaluations. The delays and deviances in the growth of the children on the unit make it essential to evaluate their functioning in life-tasks and skill areas.

The play history obtained by interviewing the child's parents or caretakers is an historical account of a child's play experiences from early years to the present. It offers a repository of information about a child's play patterns, range of affects, conflicts, fantasies, and social relationships. It offers insight into the etiology and chronicity of a child's problems as well as a baseline for treatment and parent education. A parent's level of involvement in the child's play is indicative of the quality of the parent-child relationship.

An initial play profile is performed regularly on each child to ascertain a baseline for treatment. This is a screening which evaluates a child's perceptual skill, cognitive skill, emotional/psychological status, level of sensory integration, motor development, and special interests and hobbies. The data obtained allow the staff to assign the children to the various therapeutic activities and groups on the unit.

The speech pathologist evaluates the child's speech and language development. These areas are of paramount importance in both verbal and nonverbal communication. A variety of standardized tests are used for evaluation. They provide developmental norms and refined assessments of specific psycholinguistic functions. Receptive language, expressive language, associative language, nonverbal language, articulation, fluency, voice patterns, and sentence structure are assessed within a developmental continuum. Children with language or speech problems receive an audiological evaluation because normal audition is a prerequisite to language development. A formal evaluation of the child's linguistic competence can provide a clue as to whether deficits are organic or psychogenic in origin.

The speech pathologist provides extremely valuable information for the general milieu treatment of the child. For example, a child with a receptive language impairment requires brief, direct, nonambiguous commands in order to prevent frustrations and "misbehavior" because he "wasn't listening." In fact, we have found that many children with so-called "thought disorders" have severe auditory perceptual problems.

The speech-language evaluation is particularly useful in the differential diagnosis between a schizophrenic child and language-impaired child (De Hirsch, 1967).

In addition, the speech pathologist may initiate individual speech and/or language therapy. Operant conditioning, play therapy, compensatory techniques, and developmental stimulation are some of the treatment modalities utilized.

The tests performed by the psychologist, occupational therapist, and speech pathologist complement each other and are integrated with the general clinical picture. The total evaluation strives to identify the child's physical, psychological, emotional, perceptual, academic, and developmental status in order that comprehensive, effective treatment may proceed.

ACKNOWLEDGEMENTS

This chapter was written in consultation with Niusia Shimrat, Ed.D., Chief, Child Psychology; Roberta Preisler, M.A., Assistant Psychologist; Steven Blaustein, M.S., Speech Pathologist; and Marsha Silverton, M.S.W. C.S.W. at the Mount Sinai Medical Center.

REFERENCES

Ayres, A.J. (1973). *Sensory Integration and Learning Disorders*. Los Angeles, Calif.: Western Psychological Services.

Berlin, I. (1978). Developmental issues in the psychiatric hospitalization of children. *Am. J. Psychiatry 135*:1044-1048.

Critchley, D.L., and Berlin, I.N. (1979). Day treatment of young psychotic children and their parents: Interdisciplinary issues and problems. *Child Psychia. Hum. Dev. 9*:227-237.

De Hirsch, K. (1967). Differential diagnosis between aphasic and schizophrenic language. *J. Spch. Hear. Dis. 32*:2-10.

Freud, A. (1965). *Normality and Pathology in Childhood: Assessments of Development*. New York: Int. Univ. Press.

Chapter 7

THE CHANGING ROLE OF THE PRIMARY THERAPIST ON A SHORT-TERM CHILD PSYCHIATRY INPATIENT UNIT

Jessica Hellinger-Kaslick
Marsha Silverton

There is a small body of literature that addresses the issue of psychotherapy in residential treatment and psychiatric hospitalization of children. Most authors (Bettleheim, 1966; Brodie, 1966) focus on long-term psychotherapy with children and families, and few have addressed themselves to the specific demands of a short-term psychiatric hospitalization. Historically, the literature on residential treatment and psychiatric hospitalization emphasizes the adaptation of psychoanalytic theory and technique to the treatment of the child and family (Noshpitz, 1962). This model initially resulted in an approach that treated the child as separate from the family and environment. The child was placed in a benign environment in order to allow the treatment, that is, psychotherapy or psychoanalysis, to be undertaken. This resulted in an antagonism between the primary therapist and hospital staff, when the child's psychotherapy was viewed as pristine, separate, and superior to anything accomplished by other staff in the milieu. With an increased understanding of the impact of family and environmental factors in the treatment of the child, there has been a gradual shift in attitude in residential treatment settings to viewing the child within the context of the total family unit and the therapeutic milieu. Berlin and Christ (1969) emphasize the increasing complexity of the role of the primary therapist who must be at once child therapist, family therapist, team coordinator and leader, and diagnostic synthesizer. This chapter describes the experience on a short-term (3 weeks to 3 months) child psychiatry unit where the role of the primary therapist has gradually shifted from the isolated practitioner of the psychoanalytic model to the coordinator and integrator of a team approach.

At the Mount Sinai Medical Center Child Psychiatry Inpatient Unit, the primary therapists are the child psychiatry fellows, psychiatric social workers, and occasionally other staff members. The primary therapist assumes the responsibility for the treatment of the entire case, that is, the child and significant family members. Prior to admission, the family and child are oriented to the team approach on the unit. The family is assigned to a primary therapist. Initially, some children and/or family members may experience confusion as to why they have their "sessions" with a social worker and others with a doctor. However, for the most part they do not become involved in the hierarchial conflicts which have beset the mental health field, and accept without prolonged discussion the assignment to their primary therapist. Feelings of rivalry among the children on the unit occur across all disciplines and are not related to the professional training and orientation of the staff members. One child may complain to his therapist that another child's therapist takes him out or another child is seen more frequently. The child's main concern is that he or she has one constant adult toward whom he or she can turn to mediate and be responsible for his or her existence on unit.

The role of the primary therapist on a psychiatric unit can only be understood within the context of the therapeutic milieu and a coordinated team approach. A treatment approach that encompasses and stresses the role of the professional team and the therapeutic milieu improves the morale and atmosphere on the unit. The focus on the importance of every staff member who comes into contact with the children and their families provides a therapeutic environment, and gives everyone a feeling that he or she has an impact that is valuable and significant. The primary therapist is viewed as coordinator of the therapeutic team. In order to have the team work effectively, it is important that the primary therapist have the ability to work well with members of other disciplines. The potential for staff conflicts and competitive feelings can destroy the team functioning, the impact of which is communicated readily to the child. In many instances such conflict could repeat the problems in the family which contributed to the child's need for hospitalization. Children tune into staff conflicts quickly and manipulate and play into these difficulties. It is therefore essential that there be ongoing critical evaluation of the functioning of the interdisciplinary team. Only such a coordinated team approach provides the necessary data for a complete diagnostic and therapeutic evaluation.

The primary therapist assumes the role of coordinator of these processes and integrator not only for the child and family, but for all staff members involved. Coordination of input from staff occurs during regularly scheduled case discussions where the primary therapist initiates the presentation of case material. At these meetings, specific ongoing evaluation and treatment plans are made. However, much of the day-to-day work on an inpatient child psychiatry unit is carried out through informal meetings between the therapist and other staff members.

To the extent that the primary therapist and other staff work well together, the treatment plan will be coordinated and the child's experience on the unit will be for the most part well integrated.

In short-term hospitalization, the treatment has a discrete beginning, middle, and end phase. For all children, the initial phase of treatment is devoted to the separation from the family, feelings of loss and abandonment, fears of object loss, and depression. There is a middle comfortable working phase in which the child has made an adjustment to the unit and begins to work with a therapist on issues of major concern. This short comfortable period is over as issues of disposition and discharge emerge and have to be dealt with by the therapist, the family and the child.

Initially, the child utilizes the therapist to negotiate his transition into a strange and complicated new setting. Children who have been hospitalized because of a failure in the home environment to provide adequate structure and who have not internalized their own controls often experience the structure of the unit as a safe and comfortable haven. The separation from parents may also be a frightening and difficult experience, despite the inadequacy of the home environment. Initial therapy sessions are frequently filled with ambivalent feelings about the hospital, fears of being abandoned by the family, fantasies of being punished for bad behavior, and anxiety over what will actually happen in the hospital.

The primary therapist is not only a caretaker and empathic listener, but also an authority figure for the child. He or she is viewed by the child as making and being responsible for major decisions affecting his life, such as weekend passes with family members, and ultimately, the disposition plan. Severely disturbed children easily project their own feelings of grandiosity and omnipotence. Thus, the primary therapist is frequently endowed with power and magical capacity. The child is aware that within the team structure the primary therapist is the key figure. For example, if the child or parents request a pass of someone other than the primary therapist, the staff response is "discuss it with your therapist." The child views the therapist not only in the privacy and isolated atmosphere of psychotherapy, but in the context of the complex functioning of the inpatient unit. For example, as the child observes the therapist's interactions with and responses to other children and other staff members, he or she responds in terms of his or her own sibling difficulties or in terms of his or her own identification with the other children on the unit.

It is therefore clear that the treatment of severely disturbed children requiring hospitalization must bridge the distance from the intrapsychic to the reality aspects of the child's life in order to aid the child in assessing and understanding his own experience and interactions. In keeping with this focus, the therapist on an inpatient unit makes considerable use of everyday ward experiences in psychotherapy itself. The primary therapist is privy to the details of the child's entire life situation on the unit. These details may be brought openly into the therapy and the child can begin to evaluate and understand his behavior both inside and outside the therapist's office. Just as the child's daily life cannot be separated from the psychotherapy, the therapist as a practitioner cannot be separated from the unit. In addition to dealing with everyday experiences on the unit, the therapist performs many real and concrete functions for the child. For example, the therapist brings the child to and from therapy sessions which are conducted in the therapist's offices away from the unit. The therapist thus must deal with the real issues of resistance and anxiety in the child which might prevent him or her from willingly proceeding to the session. It is not infrequent that children refuse to leave the unit for sessions. They may become aggressive and defiant with their therapist when particularly anxious. For some children, particularly in the early stages of hospitalization, the one-to-one relationship with the therapist is so frightening and threatening that the child may be fearful of leaving the unit and for a period of time must be seen within this new but comfortable surrounding. The therapist must respect the child's wishes, acknowledging the anxiety while relating in such a way so that a therapeutic alliance develops. With such a child, the therapist must approach him or her through day-to-day activities on the unit until a point is reached where the child forms an attachment and can tolerate a closer therapeutic relationship.

On a short-term service, it is particular important for the therapist to be familiar with and feel comfortable employing different therapeutic modalities. In order to evaluate the child's functioning and role within his family, the therapist needs to conduct diagnostic family sessions. This is particularly important during the early phase of hospitalization

when a treatment plan for the child and the family is being formulated.
These sessions help the therapist determine to what extent he or she
will employ individual sessions with the child and/or parents, family
sessions, milieu therapy, or a combination of these approaches. As a
psychiatric unit functions more cohesively and with greater emphasis
on the therapeutic milieu, it becomes increasingly difficult for the
therapist to treat the child's psychopathology in an isolated fashion.
Even when the therapist utilizes individual sessions with the child, the
individual treatment needs to be understood within the larger context
of the milieu and the family.

The child's behavior on the ward is usually a transferential reenactment
of the original conflicts within the family. While severe psychotic or aggressive
behavior could not be tolerated in the family or community, the milieu
provides structure and limits and attempts to help the child develop
more appropriate social behavior. Even during a short-term hospitalization, individual sessions with the child can help him to understand
what brought him to the hospital and to integrate his experiences on
the ward. The primary therapist attempts to help the child gain
insight into his family's problems through interpretation, confrontation,
and clarification. Depending on the child's age, his level of psycho-
sexual and cognitive development, as well as the fluctuations in his
emotional state, one utilizes a combination of verbal and play therapy.
The individual therapeutic approach serves to strengthen the child's
controls and appropriate defense mechanisms. The therapist does not
interpret prematurely unconscious conflict.

At the point that the primary therapist begins to understand the
child's mental life it is important that it be clarified and communicated
to other staff on an ongoing basis so that the meaning of the child's
manifest behavior can be fully appreciated and understood in terms of
the psychodynamic picture. This will ensure that logical and therapeutic
interventions can be initiated by the entire child care staff. For
example, aggressive and provocative behavior can be viewed not only
as an indicator of the child's anger but also as an indicator of underlying
anxiety. When one is attuned to such anxiety reactions, one can help
the child master such feelings. One child, after mastering his aggressive
outbursts and having made a fairly good adjustment, displayed a week
of impulse-ridden and agitated behavior. While the staff initially assumed
that the child had regressed, it became clear from the psychotherapy
sessions that the child was anxious because his parents, now divorced,
were meeting to determine a disposition plan for him. This information
became available to the general staff. The staff working closest with
this child on the milieu could make appropriate ego-supportive and
interpretative comments about his anxiety (Noshpitz, 1962). On the
night prior to the child's discharge from the hospital he was quite agitated,
wanting a "sleeping pill." He responded to reassurance and interpretative
comments made by the evening nursing staff.

When a child is seen in individual psychotherapy during short-term
hospitalization, one needs to evaluate and assess the meaning and goals
of such treatment. Clearly the treatment is not open-ended, nor will
one have the opportunity to attain an overview of long-term psychotherapy. The individual sessions offer the therapist the unique
opportunity to observe the development of transference reactions, to
evaluate the child's capacity for object relations and the prognosis for
ongoing long-term psychotherapy, and very importantly, to provide an
indication of the underlying meaning of the child's behavioral symptoms.

One child who had been hospitalized at the request of her foster
care agency had been placed in a foster home at the age of 3 until the

time of hospitalization at age 11. She had been abandoned by her mother at birth and had been raised in institutions to age 3, with some minimal contact with the natural mother. At the time of referral for hospitalization she manifested severe behavioral problems in the home and at school. Long-term residential placement was being considered. The foster family was the only family this child had known. Given the bureaucratic politics of foster care in the city in which she lived, it was clear that if this child were moved from the foster family, their contact with her would be discouraged by the foster care agency and the child would grow up in an institution, essentially isolated and alone. The hospitalization provided an evaluation of the quality of this child's relationship with her foster family, her capacity for relatedness, and a prognosis for her remaining in the family. Despite the severity of behavioral problems, the foster family was not requesting placement and the foster care agency was not in a position to adequately evaluate the underlying meaning of the child's symptoms. The agency was struck by the child's apparent disinterest and indifference to the foster family, particularly to the foster mother.

During the course of the 3-month hospitalization, the child developed a fairly intense and specific relationship with her primary therapist. This relationship differed qualitatively and quantitatively from the relationships that she established with other staff members in general. In her therapy sessions she played out intense games of hide-and-seek and turned the lights on and off. It became clear that she was reenacting early scenes reported in the history of the natural mother who had disappeared when the child was approximately age $2\frac{1}{2}$, when she subsequently moved to the foster family. The child's behavior on the unit revealed that she had the capacity to relate to people in a way which was not indiscriminate and indifferent. In the course of 3 months she had developed a fairly intense relationship with her therapist; she became rivalrous of other children for attention and gradually demonstrated interest in imitating and identifying with the therapist (a woman). While it was not possible to work through much of this early trauma during the period of hospitalization, the elaboration of this play served an important function. On the basis of her response to therapy, the foster agency agreed that the child not be placed in a residential treatment center, but rather that she be returned to her foster family and involved in an intense therapeutic relationship with a female therapist. It became clear that therapy needed to focus on issues of early separation-individuation and the abandonment of her natural mother, so that ultimately this child would be able to better utilize her attachment to the foster mother.

In addition to the work with the child, the primary therapist must maintain ongoing contact with important family members through regularly scheduled sessions. It is important to develop a therapeutic alliance with the family because without this involvement, the therapeutic contribution to the child is severely limited. It is most evident that treatment failures occur when the family cannot be engaged and they sabotage the treatment even to the point of removing the child from the hospital "against medical advice."

In a setting where a large percentage of the children come from multiproblem, economically and culturally deprived families, or families whose primary language is not English, the therapist needs to address some of the specific needs of this population. Frequently, missed or broken appointments reflect a specific resistance secondary to the family's fearfulness of the hospital as a large and overwhelming institution, their difficulty with the language barrier, and their inability to utilize effectively the particular service which is offered. Often the therapist must reach out to these patients, in a way that takes into consideration the parents' anxieties as well as their own cultural differences. The primary therapist may have to help the parent with concrete services before the parent can view the therapist as a helper. One of the first goals must be to engage the parents as allies in the treatment and evaluation process.

The first issue that most frequently surfaces revolves around the parents' feelings of guilt at having a child requiring psychiatric hospitalization. Parents state either overtly or covertly that they feel "I am a bad parent" and "I have failed in some way." Many parents project blame onto the school or someone else in the environment. However, if the primary therapist is empathic, there is a chance that the parents may eventually begin to explore their own personal problems and view the primary therapist as someone who can provide treatment for themselves.

Many parents become threatened and increasingly resistant if they are made to feel that they are being viewed as a "patient." One must begin developing the therapeutic relationship in a supportive manner, stressing to the parents that they can help the professionals to further understand *their* child. It is helpful to highlight that the multitude of questions regarding the child and the family, which are part of the history-taking process, are a way of gathering information to further understand the child and the family. The traditional child guidance approach of the social worker obtaining the history and working with the parents while the psychiatrist treats the child leads to fragmentation and does not allow for a continuous integration of the data obtained from the child and family. In contrast, the approach used at Mount Sinai, whereby the primary therapist has the direct ongoing contact with the family allows for an integration of the work done with the child and the family. The family can work with the therapist to help them with their difficulties in relation to the child.

In the beginning of hospitalization, it is common for parents to complain to the primary therapist about the physical care that the child receives on the ward, about specific staff members, and about other children. As a defense against their guilt for having a severely troubled child, parents often emphasize that the care they give at home is far superior to that on the unit. The parent perceives the staff as taking away the child and assuming a parental role. The primary therapist needs to listen to the parents' complaints, not become defensive, and understand that some of the complaints may be realistic. The parent uses the element of reality as a way of projecting his or her guilt onto the unit staff. Parents need to be reassured that the staff is not usurping the parenting responsibilities. It is critical to create an atmosphere where parents understand that the orientation is not to place "blame" on anyone for the problems. In fact it is often beneficial to tell parents beforehand that their child will have innumerable complaints and that the adjustment period will be difficult for both parents and child.

One 10-year-old boy was admitted for severe learning problems and multiple behavior problems at home and school. The mother was emphatic about her belief that the school was responsible for her son's problems. She was angry and abusive to the teacher and principal. She denied any problems in the home environment. As she began to trust the primary therapist, she confided that she had had an extramarital affair, was not certain if this was her husband's child, and during her pregnancy had purchased some medication to induce abortion. When this medication did not work, she decided to follow through with the pregnancy. She was frightened that the medication had damaged her child and that his symptoms and hospitalization were a punishment for her wrongdoing. This mother became increasingly overwhelmed with what she considered "her secret burden." Her complaints were clearly a projection of this guilt. After the mother could speak more directly of her guilt, she related more realistically to her son's problems, her own behavior became more appropriate, and she was able to begin work on discharge planning.

In addition to work with parents, the primary therapist often must become involved with multiple significant family members. A 7-year-old girl was admitted to the inpatient unit following a history of behavioral problems at home and at school, suicidal ideation, and one suicidal gesture which included sitting on the window ledge at school threatening to jump. The family constellation included divorced parents and a new mate for each parent. There was a long-standing history of marital discord prior to the divorce which had occurred when the patient was 4 years old. The patient lived with her mother for approximately 8 months and then was shifted to the father because of the mother's own personal problems and inability to handle the child. This young girl lived alone with her father in a small apartment until 5 months prior to hospitalization when the father's girlfriend moved into the home. Around the same time, the mother's boyfriend moved in with the mother. The two sets of family members were antagonistic to each other and refused to meet jointly. Sessions with the two sets of family members enabled them to understand that the child was placed in the middle of the many ongoing unresolved battles. They were helped to understand that the sudden addition of mates caused the child to panic about possibly losing the attention of each parent. The primary therapist stressed the importance of working out a structured plan so that the child would know exactly how much time she would spend with each parent. One of the parental sets (paternal) was able to utilize the sessions and deal with their relationship to each other and to the child. There were many family sessions that included the patient and her primary family unit of father and stepmother. The focus of these sessions enabled the patient to feel that she belonged to this new unit.

The question of disposition after discharge from the unit needs to be dealt with by the child, the therapist, and the family almost from the beginning of hospitalization. In view of the primary therapist's unique understanding of both the child and family, he or she has a major input into the team decision of formulating the disposition plan. A goal of hospitalization is to decide whether the child will be able to return to the family with the built-in support of special schooling, day treatment, psychotherapy, medication, or a combination of these. In certain circumstances, because of the severity of the child's or the family's psychopathology, the child may require a period of continued separation from the family in a residential treatment center. When the primary therapist assumes the total responsibility for a case, he or she initiates and follows through on the specifics of the discharge plan. This may entail making the referrals for residential treatment or special school, the scheduling of admission interviews, as well as preparing the child and family. Traditionally, discharge planning on the psychiatric inpatient unit has been the function of the social worker. *When this crucial function is assumed by the primary therapist, the process of discharge planning is brought directly into the treatment and provides*

*an avenue by which the child and family can experience and work
through their feelings about the impending plans.*

For the child and family this last phase of hospitalization is devoted
to feelings of loss and separation from the unit and the staff as well
as anxiety about returning home and/or another setting. The parents
often have difficulty separating from the primary therapist and the
unit. For many of them, the unit takes on a protective and parenting
role because they are needy and infantile themselves. Some parents
state outright that they wish they could be admitted to the unit. For
some families the termination process involves preparing the child to
return to the environment in which he or she originally experienced
overwhelming difficulty. An important goal of hospitalization is to
build supports into the home environment to prevent the child and
family from becoming overwhelmed once again. Some families continue
outpatient psychotherapy with the same therapist, usually on a once-
a-week basis. Often a child may be placed in a special class which is
geared to deal with specific problems such as emotional difficulties,
neurological impairments, learning disability, or low-level intellectual
functioning. The outpatient psychotherapy experience does not have
the same intensity that occurs during the period of hospitalization and
may therefore make this a difficult transition for parent and child.

When children from the inpatient unit go on to long-term residential
treatment centers, they leave the family as well as the familiar hospital
environment. Children who often experience the plan as a rejection
or another abandonment must deal with their anger and anxiety about
going to another unknown environment. They often do not understand
why they cannot stay on the unit indefinitely. Parental feelings of
ambivalence must be handled sensitively at each step or else the parents
may sabotage the plans for residential treatment. In many parents,
underlying feelings of anger and guilt are projected onto the child and
the staff. In some cases, the primary therapist can interpret this
defensive maneuver unless it is felt that the parent needs such a
primitive defensive structure to prevent overwhelming anxiety.

A 32-year-old divorced mother experienced a period of depression
when long-term residential placement for her child was suggested. She
required a combination of regular psychotherapy sessions and medication.
The child's need for continued residential treatment reawakened her
early feelings of abandonment by her own mother, multiple separations,
her own insecurity, lack of nurturance, and guilt regarding her inability
to provide a home for her child. Interpretation and clarification of the
meaning of these feelings within the context of this mother's own
developmental history enabled her to feel less overwhelmed, less guilty,
and more in control of her own life and decisions. Ultimately, she was
able to follow through on placement plans.

For the child, the family, and the therapist, the experience of a
short-term hospitalization offers a very intense, time-limited venture.
The hospitalization, with its own built-in stages, provides the momentum
for treatment which could not possibly be sustained on a long-term
basis. There is a quality to working with children and families in a
short-term psychiatric hospital unit that makes it extraordinarily
demanding emotionally. However, it offers the child, the family, and
the therapist a very gratifying and rewarding experience that is often
lifesaving.

REFERENCES

Barker, P. (1974). *The Residential Psychiatric Treatment of Children*. New York: Wiley.

Berlin, I. (1978). Developmental issues in the psychiatric hospitalization of children. *Am. J. Psychiatry 135(9)*: 1044-1048.

Berlin, I., and Christ, A. (1969). The unique role of the child psychiatry trainee on an inpatient or day care unit. *J. Am. Acad. Child Psychiatry 8*: 247-258.

Bettleheim, B. (1966). Training the child care worker in a residential center. *Am. J. Orthopsychiatry 36*: 694-705.

Brodie, R. (1966). Some aspects of psychotherapy in a residential treatment center. *Am. J. Orthopsychiatry 36(4)*: 712-719.

Brunstetter, R. (1969). Status, role and the function of supervision in the residential treatment center for children. *J. Am. Acad. Child Psychiatry 8*: 259-271.

Harrison, S., McDermott, J., and Chethek, M. (1969). Residential treatment of children: The psychotherapist-administrator. *J. Am. Acad. Child Psychiatry 8*: 385-410.

Hirschberg, J. (1953). The role of education in the treatment of emotionally disturbed children through planned ego development. *Am. J. Orthopsychiatry 23(44)*: 684-690.

Noshpitz, J. (1962). Notes on the theory of residential treatment. *J. Am. Acad. Child Psychiatry 1*: 284-296.

Redl, F. (1959). The concept of a therapeutic milieu. *Am. J. Orthopsychiatry 29*: 721-736.

Szurek, S.A., Berlin, I.N., and Boatman, M. (1971). *Inpatient Care for the Psychotic Child*. The Langley Porter Child Psychiatry Series, Vol. 5. Palo Alto, Calif.: Science and Behavior Books.

Chapter 8

THE FAMILY OF THE HOSPITALIZED CHILD

Lois Shein

The psychiatric evaluation and treatment of severely disturbed children requires a basic commitment to family involvement by the treating staff. As described in the previous chapter, children cannot be assessed or treated in a vacuum and must be seen within the context of the family. Parents need to be actively involved with the staff at the screening interview, treatment in the hospital, and during the planning stages for posthospital treatment. They are the ones who ultimately bear the responsibility for what happens to their child.

Parents who are faced with a decision about hospitalizing their disturbed child feel frightened and vulnerable. The vast majority feel guilty about their child's illness and this is often intensified by the act of hospitalization. They feel that they have failed in their parental role, that their child will resent them for having been placed in the hospital, and that the professional staff will prove to be better parents. One must be constantly attuned to these feelings.

Some parents readily express their guilt and assume blame for their child's problems, others project the guilt, and still others deny that there is a problem. The staff members need to be aware of their own reactions to the parents. It can be very difficult to deal with the parents who use the defenses of denial and projection. The manifest behavior of blaming others for the child's problems often arouses anger and frustration in the staff. "If the staff feelings are not resolved they reveal themselves to parents, who, in turn become defensive" (Magnus, 1974). It is important for all staff members to recognize and empathize with this underlying guilt and understand the parental reaction as defensive. False reassurance should not be given because it simply intensifies guilt.

The staff must guard against overidentifying with the child and blaming the parents for the child's problem; this is not an infrequent problem in the treatment of children and their families. Many parents' efforts at parenting are stymied by their own pathology, defects in their child, or overwhelming social conditions. The staff must be careful not to be judgmental, but instead to try to understand not only what life is like for the child, but for the parents as well.

Many of the children hospitalized on the inpatient service at Mount Sinai Medical Center come from families of low socioeconomic status with all the concomitant problems of a ghetto population. Many come

53

from single-parent homes where family life is disorganized and chaotic.
The parents are often overwhelmed by the demands of day-to-day living.
They have few supports available to them in the community, and only
limited internal coping mechanisms. Many are themselves emotionally
disturbed, have poor impulse control, are abusive and/or abused, and
suffer from depression, alcoholism, or drug addiction. When parents,
for example, are not keeping appointments, the staff should not dismiss
them as disinterested. Instead, they need to assess the parents'
external and internal strengths and weaknesses, and assess the reason
for the apparent lack of interest. An alternate approach may reinvolve
the parent more actively. "Not every parent can be brought to accept
the sharing role in treatment. However, the institution should continue
to involve parents until all efforts have indeed proved futile...If the
parents simply are not interested or able to help, we must still treat
them with dignity and respect" (Magnus, 1974). For example, the
mother of a retarded aggressive child, herself retarded, did not keep
appointments with the primary therapist. The therapist arranged for
weekly contact by telephone, and encouraged the mother to continue
to visit the child on weekends.

From the pont of referral, the staff must be aware of the parents'
feelings and attitudes. Even overtly "rejecting" parents need to be
actively involved in the process throughout. They should be involved
in the decision about whether or not to hospitalize their child and
should receive a clear explanation from the professional staff as to why
hospitalization is being recommended. The parents need to visit the
facility where their child will be, understand what can be offered to
the child and family, and meet the staff to whom they are entrusting
their child. If the parents' role is usurped by the professionals, the
hospitalization may prove intolerable for one or both parents, and the
child may be removed precipitously, with the hospital experience being
destructive for the child and family. "It is painful for the family to
hospitalize a child. Some of its guilt and ambivalence is lessened when
the family can be active in the treatment process" (Kemp, 1971). The
treatment process begins with the first contact between the hospital
staff and the family. Even though clinically, hospitalization for the
child may be indicated, if the parent is not ready to accept this, a
period of outpatient contact is necessary to prepare the parents and
child for separation and minimize its deleterious effects.

L., a 9-year-old boy, was referred by the school on an emergency
basis because of fire-setting and sitting on window ledges. He was
admitted immediately with the mother's approval. The following day
the father appeared at the hospital insisting his son be released as
he saw no reason for the child to be hospitalized. The staff tried to
help the father understand his son's needs, but it was obviously too
late; the father felt that his role as a parent had been usurped by his
wife and the hospital staff. In contrast to the above case, D., a
9-year-old boy known to the outpatient department for several years,
was brought for inpatient admission by his father while his mother was
herself a psychiatric patient in the hospital. The child had markedly
regressed during the mother's hospitalization and demonstrated serious
pathology. The mother was adamantly opposed to having her son
hospitalized. Rather than admit the boy with only the father's permission,
the staff met with the mother's therapist who helped the mother understand the need for hositalizing her son; within several hours, the
mother reluctantly agreed to speak with the unit staff, visited the unit,
and agreed to admit her son. During the child's hospitalization,
because she did not see the hospital as threatening authority who wanted

to take her child away, she was able to work cooperatively with the primary therapist. In fact, the experience was a sufficiently positive one for her and her child that at discharge she agreed to long-term residential treatment, something which she had previously opposed. Only by demonstrating at the outset that she remain the parent, with all the rights and responsibilities towards her child, could she agree with this plan.

These case illustrations highlight the importance of parental involvement beginning at the admission process. Professionals often feel pressured when a child appears to be in imminent danger. Rescue fantasies, so common in the child care field, lead to a response to offer an immediate protective environment for the child. However, if just the needs of the child are considered and not the needs of the parents, the success not only of treatment, but of the hospitalization itself, is questionable. In the long run, the hospital cannot "rescue" the child without parental cooperation. It is far more productive to work with a resistant family prior to admission than to have the family discharge the child precipitously. Certainly if the child is in serious danger and the parents continue to refuse treatment, the professional staff does have the responsibility to involve the authority of the court or the Division of Children's Services.

Once the child is admitted, parents must continue to feel that they have the ultimate responsibility for all decisions that are made regarding their child. No treatment can be successful without the parents' agreement. Therefore, the staff needs to share, in language the parents can understand, results of all evaluations, psychiatric, psychological, and medical. From the outset, the parents need to be engaged in a working relationship with the primary therapist and other hospital staff. They need to meet regularly with the therapist and be directly involved in the treatment process.

In the child guidance model, parents and children are seen by different therapists, and the parents' contact with the person to whom they entrust their child is minimal. This is not a viable treatment plan. In order to foster a working alliance with the entire family, it is essential that one therapist assume responsibility for that family. From the parents' point of view, it means that they no longer get information about their child secondhand, but instead can discuss their concerns directly with the person who knows their child best. They feel more connected to decisions about their child's treatment. The therapist who sees the complex family interactions firsthand can thus evaluate the strengths and weaknesses within the entire family system. When working with the family, the therapist must constantly guard against overidentifying with either the child or the parents. This is more easily accomplished when the therapist assumes treatment responsibilities for both parents and child. "When the worker sees the whole family as a client, he is not likely to always see the child as a victim requiring rescue or the parents as overwhelmed, and in need of relief from a tyranical child. He will see the interlocking strengths and weaknesses of every member of the family" (Moss, 1968).

The designated patient is not necessarily the most disturbed member of the family, but may instead be the one who demonstrates behavior that the family system or community can least tolerate (Guerin, 1976). A family-focused approach does not necessarily mean that the family as a whole is seen as the treatment unit. It means instead that the entire family is evaluated. The assessment of the individual members' needs and availability and the family interrelationships results in a treatment plan for the family members as well as for the designated patient.

The therapist must remember that the parents are not "patients" and that they are coming on behalf of their child and not for their own symptoms or problems. Many parents, from the outset or during the course of the child's hospitalization, do recognize their own need for treatment, but to begin by putting the parents in a patient role often creates a situation which the parents cannot tolerate and from which they withdraw. At the point of the child's admission to the hospital, parents, because of their feelings of inadequacy and vulnerability, are concerned about being seen as disturbed or as causative factors in their child's problems. They need support, acceptance, and reassurance. If one quickly shifts the focus from the child to the parents or to family problems, the parents' guilt intensifies and they become more defensive. The shift to the family's problems needs to be forestalled until the parents feel less vulnerable and are more capable of looking at themselves and the total family system.

E., a 9-year-old diabetic boy, was hospitalized because of severe behavioral difficulties at home and a refusal to follow the medical regime for his diabetes. It was clear at the point of evaluation that the family relationships were grossly impaired and that severe marital difficulties impaired the parents' ability to deal with E. effectively. The parents, however, were not ready to examine their role in E.'s difficulties. They focused all their thoughts on their concerns for E. and were very critical of the unit staff. The primary therapist listened to them empathically and conveyed a feeling that the staff members did not consider themselves better parents. When the parents felt accepted and less vulnerable, they became less defensive and began to discuss their serious marital difficulties. Only then could they shift their focus from E. onto the underlying difficulties of the family. If the primary therapist had attempted this earlier, she would have heightened the parents' resistance.

Therapeutic planning must take into account the needs of the child, the parents, and other family members. "It is our obligation to the family, once we admit its child to the hospital, to invest in the family, and to use this opportunity to strengthen and improve the functioning of all its members" (Kemp, 1971). Even though the child is the designated patient, the treatment plan for the other family members must be as carefully and thoughtfully arrived at as the plan for the child. During the initial period of hospitalization a variety of family meetings should be conducted in order to assess the family interaction and the most crucial family issues which need to be addressed during the period of hospitalization.

It is important to plan some individual sessions with the parents in order to discuss treatment plans and recommendations and to enable them to deal with their guilt and other feelings about themselves and their disturbed child. Parents who continue to feel overwhelming guilt regarding their child are stymied in their ability to make decisions about the child's treatment and future planning. Many parents resist meeting individually with the therapist because of the worry that they will be blamed and held responsible for their child's problems. At times the parents' psychopathology precludes a therapeutic involvement. These parents may be more able to participate in a therapeutic process via a group situation or family sessions as the main treatment modality or as a prelude to individual sessions. The primary therapist, in conjunction with the other members of the miniteam, needs to determine the most therapeutic approach.

D., a 12-year-old boy, was hospitalized because of severe behavioral problems. His mother appeared rejecting and disinterested, and kept none of the individual appointments offered to her. However, with encouragement from the staff, she did begin attending the parent's group. It became clear in the group that her guilt, vulnerability, and anxiety were masked by a rejecting and punitive facade. Her therapist, who was a co-leader in the group, could empathize with her feelings, give appropriate support and thus establish a relationship which allowed her to speak with the therapist without fear of being blamed or seen as a bad mother. This approach, plus an accepting attitude, encouraged her to become engaged in a relationship on behalf of her child.

Even in situations where ongoing individual treatment for the parents is the treatment of choice, family sessions should be conducted with the child and family. A series of family sessions are critical in order to assess the family's functioning and interrelationships. Family sessions should involve the total nuclear family and, where appropriate, extended family members as well. If this isn't possible, the child should be interviewed at least with the significant adults. Observations of a family in action often clarify family dynamics more effectively than verbal descriptions by other family members. The assessment of the family includes not only diagnosing pathology, but also diagnosing strengths and resources within the family. The nature of the strengths and resources often determines the progress that the family and child can make during the hospitalization and after discharge.

Home visits enable the staff to observe the family's environment. Unfortunately, because of distances, this is not always practical. When parents do not keep regular appointments, or when the situation remains unclear after several sessions, a home visit can engage an absent member or clarify the family dynamics. Most parents are quite pleased to have the staff make a home visit. When a family is to be visited at home, the child accompanies the staff from the hospital so he or she can participate in the interview.

Many children who have had difficulties prior to hospitalization have often been actively involved with another agency. This agency needs to be kept informed during the child's hospitalization because the referring agency often implements the plan at discharge. When a parent has a working relationship with someone in another agency, that alliance is fostered in the tratment and planning for the child and family. Outside therapists are invited to case discussions and to visit with the child, particularly if the child is to resume treatment with them upon discharge. If the parent continues an involvement with the referring agency, the primary therapist maintains some regular contact with the parent in order to coordinate the child's treatment during hospitalization.

In addition to the individual and family approaches, a parent or family group is a useful therapeutic tool in engaging parents and helping them deal with the impact of their child's hospitalization. Parents require the additional support of others who are experiencing similar problems and anxieties about their hospitalized child. They are often concerned about whether or not they did the right thing, they wonder whether their child will be angry with them, and they don't know what and how to tell other people. In the group, they can share feelings and discuss these issues with parents who are experiencing similar concerns as well as with those who have made some resolution. They thus feel less isolated and can deal with some of their conflicts. One must remember that this is a period of heightened vulnerability for parents who need to be offered multiple supports.

Parents of hospitalized children often seek each other out during visiting hours for support and reassurance. The parents' group at Mount Sinai Medical Center, for example, which is co-led by a social worker, nurse, and child psychiatry fellow, was the outgrowth of the nursing staff's observations that parents were drawn to each other during visiting hours. This informal meeting led to a weekly meeting which many parents attend regularly. The group focuses on common concerns and problems. Some of the issues discussed include the parents' feelings about their child's hospitalization, the children's day-to-day living in the hospital, problems or complaints about the staff or unit policies, their own personal problems which they wish to share, and their concerns and worries about discharge. The group therapists need to strike a balance between giving information and dealing with the feelings aroused by the child's hospitalization. The usefulness and support derived from the group experience can best be illustrated by the following vignette from a group session.

Mrs. V. was a regular and active member of the group. At Mrs. V.'s last meeting, Mrs. D. thanked her for her support during the initial period of hospitalization, and acknowledged that without it, she wasn't sure she could have permitted her child to stay. Mrs. V.'s response was to tell Mrs. D. that she was now in a position to help someone else going through the initial adjustment period which, in fact, Mrs. D. had already begun doing with a couple new to the group. It was quite clear from this exchange that both parents experienced and valued the support which they derived from other parents in the group.

In addition to the planned contact with the primary therapist and via groups, parents have frequent in-person (during visiting hours) and telephone contact with other unit staff, particularly the nursing and child care staff. These contacts need to be supportive of the treatment plan for the parents, and are an important source of information. It is crucial that the primary therapist and the other staff share information regularly, not only in relation to the child, but also in relation to the parents. In order to maximize the therapeutic effort, all staff must be aware of what is happening in a family, what particular concerns the parents have, and how to address these concerns in a coordinated and productive manner.

Parents must be involved in the treatment of their child. The commitment to a family-focused approach is imperative at all stages of the child's hospitalization if one is to begin to be successful in the treatment of severely disturbed children.

REFERENCES

Black, J. (1967). Group therapy of parents who have children in residential or day care treatment. *J. Asthma Res.* 4:251-252.

Guerin, P.J. (1976). *Family Therapy: Theory and Practice.* New York: Gardner Press.

Heiting, K. (1971). Involving parents in residential treatment of children. *Children Today* 18:162-167.

Kemp, C.J. (1971). Family treatment within the milieu of a residential treatment center. *Child Welfare* 50:229-235.

Kysar, J.E. (1968). Reactions of professionals to disturbed children and their parents. *Arch. Gen. Psychiatry* 19:562-570.

Levy, L.P. (1977). Services to parents of children in a psychiatric hospital. *Soc. Casework* 00:204-213.

Magnus, R.A. (1974). Parent involvement in residential treatment programs. *Children Today* 3:25-27.

Moss, S.A. (1968). Integration of the family into the child placement process. *Children Today* 15:219-224.
Reidy, J.J. (1962). Family treatment approaches: An approach to family-centered treatment in a state institution. *Am. J. Orthopsychiatry* 32:133-141.

Chapter 9

THERAPEUTIC ACTIVITIES FOR THE HOSPITALIZED CHILD

Robyn Abramson

Latency-age children have to accomplish several tasks. They need to master a variety of impulses and begin to sublimate them into socially acceptable forms, they need to further develop their cognitive skills and continue the process of mastering the environment, and they need to increase their bonds in peer groups (Sarnoff, 1976; Scheidlinger 1966, and Shapiro and Perry, 1976). The child's developmental progression is facilitated by play, games, and activities, integral functions of a child's daily life (Erikson, 1977; Goldenson and Hartley, 1963; Kaplan and Kaplan, 1976; Lowenfled, 1967; Piaget, 1962; Sutton and Smith, 1974). When a child engages in an activity he or she has the opportunity to develop motor, cognitive, and perceptual skills, to learn a wide range of behaviors and emotional responses, and to explore his or her interests.

In psychotherapy, play affords the child opportunities for self-expression and communication. It allows for tension discharge, sublimation, symbolism, and mastery of intrapsychic conflicts. (Abramson, Hoffman, and Johns, 1979; Slavson and Schiffner, 1975; Schaeffer, 1975). For many children it is easier to communicate and express their feelings nonverbally than through speech. For the early latency-age child, puppetry, doll play, and drawing provide a technique for dramatizing and externalizing intrapsychic issues. For the older latency-age child, board games may become catalysts for communication and interpersonal relationships. At all times, play, games, and activities are active experiences, and their focus on productivity and participation offer intrinsic satisfaction for the child: To cultivate those skills necessary to fulfill life roles.

Greenacre (1971) points out that disturbances in the play of early childhood can lead to subsequent difficulties. Familial disturbances may interfere with social development leading to solitary play, a lack of structured play may lead to poor impulse control, and a paucity of self-expressive/creative activities may cause an undeveloped sense of self. Play cannot follow a progressive developmental course through maturational pressures alone; it requires input from the environment, that is, via play, games, and activities with family and friends.

Emotionally disturbed children have specific problems both in the pattern and quality of their play and activities as well as in their social relationships. The developmental lines of egocentricity to

61

companionship, body to play, and play to work seem to be primary targets of friction (A. Freud, 1965). Many of the children have no friends and are isolated from their peer group. Their unsocialized behavior, particularly their aggressiveness, inhibits the development of companionships. These children are unable to repress their primitive impulses. Even though most are of school age they can not engaged in latency-age games. Rarely do they have hobbies or special interests. Their play skills are limited and lack creative expression. Instead, they crave sensory stimulation via water and sand play, fingerpainting, and gross motor games; these are preschool activities, and the developmental deviance of these play patterns reflects the disequilibrium of their growth.

Their play differs from normal children more in its quality than content (Schaefer, 1975). The play of a normal child may show many hostile themes toward parents but with less intensity of feelings. The play of emotionally disturbed children is usually more variable and unpredictable. An autistic child's play may be repetitive, ritualistic, dissociated, and bizarre. An anxious and fearful child's play may be very much inhibited.

Many of the children admitted to the inpatient unit come from very deprived environments. They have had a paucity of play experiences growing up. Thus, their stay at the hospital is often the first time they have toys and playmates. Play, games, and activities are well integrated into the structure of the unit and used by all disciplines in the evaluation and treatment of the children and their families with the therapeutic activities staff providing consultation.

The major thrust of the therapeutic activities staff is to develop and provide a program (conjointly with other other staff) of group, individual, and parent-child activities based on the developmental and psychotherapeutic needs of the child and family. Much of the background to the program is based on the work of Llorens and Rubin (1967), Ayres (1973), and Slavson and Schiffer (1975). Most of the remediation occurs within the context of group activities because the children who are hospitalized not only have cognitive and perceptual deficits, but also have severe deficits in their social relationships and peer group inter-actions. Thus all groups provide an avenue to mastering particular skills and to improving social interactions.

In order to ensure that the activities are geared to the develop-mental and psychotherapeutic needs of the children, each child is discussed weekly by all team members. The child's placement in a variety of groups is the result of the observations by the various staff, the occupational therapists' play interview, as well as the existing composition of the groups. Throughout the hospitalization, there is an ongoing evaluation of the appropriateness of the group placements.

Each child is expected to attend a number of structured groups a week. These groups are well integrated into the child's schedule and the unit structure. Some of the groups focus on helping the children master and develop their cognitive, perceptual, motor, and social skills, while others focus on helping the child deal with a variety of intrapsychic and interpersonal problems. The groups which focus on developing cognitive and other skills are usually conducted by the occupational therapist or the activity therapist conjointly with a nursing staff member. The psychotherapeutic groups are conducted by a variety of staff members. The data obtained from such groups are incorporated into the discussions about the child. After each group there is usually a "wrap-up" session by the staff participating in the group. There is a weekly meeting at which time the various psychothera-

peutic groups are discussed in order to provide feedback and supervision for staff.

Some children are unable to participate in group activities because
of severe behavioral difficulties, severe anxiety in group situations,
lack of an appropriate peer group, and so on. Individual activity
sessions prior to assignment to a group allow the child to develop a
sense of trust, experience positive reinforcement and develop a sense
of mastery and achievement.

Other children, particularly very young or severely developmentally
disabled children require individual remediation. The individual program
is geared to the developmental requirements of the child. The teachers
engage the children in a tutorial program during which time the child
is involved in skill exercises to help reach grade level. The therapeutic
activities staff engage the children in selected activities for perceptual
remediation and general cognitive stimulation. The nursing staff
encourages activities which improve peer interaction, daily life skills,
and general appropriate functioning. In this way, the child may
progress developmentally at his or her own rate.

A variety of activities are employed. Obstacle courses, play-all
ball, Twister, rockboats, block building, and Simon-says help develop
gross motor skills and *body self-awareness*. Candy-land, Sesame
Street, Balloon Game, Curious George, and Missing Match-ups are
games which help develop basic visual perceptual skills such as learning
colors, numbers, letters, matching, and sorting. Cutting, tracing,
pasting and puzzles all help develop *fine motor skills*. Water play,
sand play, Play-doh, and finger painting provide *sensory stimulation*
and provide activities to help develop *parallel play skills*. Storytelling,
picture naming, card games, checkers, and backgammon help develop
concrete thinking processes such as learning cause and effect, rules
of games, right and wrong, and increasing general fund of knowledge.
Some children require aid in their *activities of daily living*. They may
need help with their dressing, toileting, eating, and so on.

Rocking is an activity which may be helpful to autistic, psychotic,
withdrawn-depressed, and hyperactive-agitated children. Autistic
children often crave the vestibular stimulation provided by a play-all
or rockboat. Fast rhythmic rocking may facilitate increased activity
in the withdrawn child and slow rhythmic rocking may calm and soothe
an agitated child. Whenever rocking is employed, the staff has to be
aware of overstimulation leading to loss of balance, head control, vertigo,
dizziness, nausea, alarm, or change in cardiac rhythm.

The following are a few clinical illustrations:

O. was a 10-year-old, bilingual retarded girl whose play skills
were limited. Her home environment was overstimulating in many ways,
yet wanting in appropriate developmental stimulation. By observing
her play, games, and activities, the staff concluded that O. had the
potential to learn. Individual sessions were structured to help increase
her general fund of knowledge and develop basic social and perceptual
skills. Lotto games were used to develop form constancy and stimulate
expressive language skills. During all activities of daily living, the
staff reinforced the names of concrete and familiar objects. Initially,
O. utilized only nonverbal gestures to communicate her needs and
wants. Before discharge, her communication skills had progressed
significantly and her level of play improved. Group activities and
experimentation with a variety of media enabled O. to progress from
imitative to parallel play and demonstrate a spontaneous involvement
and pleasure in her daily activities.

L., a 10-year-old child, was admitted because of suicidal gestures

and refusal to go to school. Her play history revealed a pattern of
solitary play and sadistic handling of dolls. Treatment goals focused
on using group experiences to decrease her social isolation. Fantasy
play with dolls enabled the therapist to explore with the child her
aggressive feelings.

A., a 7-year-old abused child, was so frightened of his environment
that he was unable to make contact. In the playroom, he would rigidly
sit with his arms folded; when the therapist tried to encourage his
involvement in activities, he would begin to tremble and utter a meek
"no." Before he could participate in activities, he had to be sure he
would not be abused by the staff.

As a final example, B., an 11-year-old depressed child, was
isolated and withdrew from activities when first admitted to the hospital.
Through participation in a drawing group, he was able to discover
his artistic talents and increase his self-esteem. After discharge he
joined an art class and set up a studio in his basement.

The following are brief descriptions of the *groups* and their *specific
goals*.

Skills groups are developmental task groups. They promote development of cognitive and social skills to enable the child to function in
academic and everyday situations. Graded activity experiences help
the child develop specific skills. For example, a child who has poor
or underdeveloped social skills will first engage in a parallel play
group, then a project group, then a cooperative group. Skills groups
are divided developmentally into three sections.

The basic skills group is for children functioning on a 4 to 6 year-
old level in preacademic skills areas. These children often have
problems in visual perception (visual motor skills, figure ground
discrimination, form constancy, and spatial relationships). They may
concomitantly demonstrate short attention span, low frustration tolerance,
and hyperactivity. Their egocentricity may prevent them from
functioning in a parallel play environment. The basic skills group is
geared to dealing with individual needs within a group context. Simple
repetitive tasks, such as tracing, cutting, pasting, and coloring
facilitate skill learning. M. was a 6-year-old child who came to the
hospital not knowing how to cut with a scissors; he used a cylindrical
grasp as his dominant prehension pattern. With formal teaching and
training M. was able to acquire the appropriate physical and perceptual
skills. His short attention span was increased through the use of a
kitchen timer and reward system.

The intermediate skills group is for children functioning on a 7 to
9 year-old level. These children do not lack specific skills but have
difficulty performing. For many, a low self-concept, strong dependency
needs, and/or a psychotic thinking process may interfere with their
functioning. The group leader helps the child develop adaptive
ego functions. For example, a child who has fluid ego boundaries may
learn to use obsessive defenses in order to engage in an activity and
have a complete end product. J., a 9-year-old anxious child, was
frightened of activities because of his rigid superego structure and his
fear of losing control. He felt he was a bad and worthless person.
With support from the therapist, activities were structured in order to
avoid potentially regressive situations. J. began to enjoy playing and
developed a hobby of making paper airplanes. Building airplanes
helped him master his feelings of vulnerability and abandonment which
stemmed from his mother's many unexplained airplane trips.

In the intermediate skills group, interaction is characterized by minimal cooperation and competition around short-term tasks. Individual activities are used to strengthen motor performance and latency-age board games are used to stimulate group awareness and further cognitive functioning.

The advanced skills group is for children functioning on a 9- to 11-year-old level. These children have mastered basic skills and are able to function somewhat independently in activities as well as in a social context. The goals of the group are to develop those cognitive skills needed to problem-solve, organize, follow directions, and be creative in an independent manner. The group promotes group inter-action skills so that the children engage in cooperative relationships. A secondary goal is to develop activity interests which may be continued outside the planned environment of the group. The group leader assumes a more passive role than in the other groups. He or she facilitates cooperation and offers supervision when necessary. Board games such as monopoly, charades, "supersandwich," and group projects such as baking and murals are used to facilitate group goals.

M., an 11-year-old boy whose cognitive and social skills were age-appropriate, had difficulties with his spontaneity. His low self-concept and conflicts about competitive drives inhibited his function-ing. During a structured board game, M. would at times withdraw from the group when competitive issues would arise. The therapist would interpret the defensive nature of this withdrawal at the moment it occurred and encouraged him to join the group activity. Ongoing positive reinforcement for participating in a group activity helped develop his self-confidence. As M. became less fragile, he experienced a game loss as less threatening to his ego and was able to begin to enjoy group games.

Community cooking is conducted once a week. This is a time when the children help prepare an evening dinner. This is a reality-based activity where the children learn the rules of cooking, the "ABC's" of nutrition, and very importantly, principles of cooperative activity.

Girls' group is a discussion group for preadolescent girls. They are given an opportunity to discuss developmental issues such as changing body image, sexuality, grooming, hygiene, heterosexual relationships, and authority relationships. The particular topic and format is geared to the developmental level and psychopathology of the particular group. Often, structured didactic sessions are provided to decrease potentially stimulating experiences. The girls often feel more comfortable discussing feelings, worries, and anxieties in this group than in the heterosexual groups or individual sessions. Group members may become catalysts for each other. For example, one 10-year-old abused child openly spoke about her parent's physical abuse. A group discussion of this issue led an 11-year-old sexually overstimu-lated child to speak about her fears of physical contact and anger at her mother's neglect. Both girls were able to be empathic and support each other as well as develop a trusting relationship with the female leaders of the group. They strengthened their own identity through a positive identification with the female role models. Sex play on the unit is another frequent group topic. Peer pressure often reinforces appropriate behavior more effectively than reprimands from the staff. In fact, on a small unit sex play is a recurrent problem. The staff have to curtail this as much as possible and help the children work through underlying motivations, fears, and anxieties about sexuality.

Cub Scouts is a club for the latency-age boys. Formal meetings are conducted weekly by a cub master and den mother who are both members of the unit staff. Meetings are structured to emphasize

individual achievement and cooperation. The children engage in
scouting activities such as knot-tying, physical fitness, conservation,
health care, and conduct codes. The children wear uniforms as a way
of recognizing their commitment to the pack and earn merit badges
as a way of building self-concept. The activities stress individual
achievement and help develop feelings of self-worth.

M., a 10-year-old boy, became involved in the Cub Scouts where
he developed his leadership potential and formed a positive identification
with his peer group. During the day, M. would refer to his scouting
activities and spontaneously organize the other boys into the pack for
a meeting. He would review and teach the conduct codes and made
temporary hats and badges. This occurred when he felt most vulnerable
and disorganized. The Cub Scouts had a reorganizing influence on
him, allowing him a time to develop his assets.

Mooving and Grooving is a group for children (primarily the
younger ones) with soft neurological signs, such as apraxia, form and
space dysfunction, tactile defensiveness, and vestibular dysfunction
(Ayres, 1973). These children often are hyperactive and impulsive
and have low frustration tolerance and a poor body image. The
group's focus helps the children receive, filter, and process all types
of sensory stimuli in order to help them make adaptive responses to
the environment. They have the opportunity to develop and master
gross motor skills and develop creativity through movement. The
activities selected incorporate a neurophysiological frame of reference
(Ayres, 1973) and dance therapy techniques. Each group begins by
providing tactile and vestibular inputs via rolling on a mat, spinning
toys, and scooter board activities. This stimulation promotes the
development of immature sensory systems, so that higher level functions
may emerge (bilateral integration, visual perception, motor planning).
The session proceeds to activities which inhibit primitive reflex
patterns such as asymmetric tonic neck reflex and tonic labyrinthine
reflex via the scooter board and gymnastics. Bilateral sensori-motor
integration and the refinement of spatial perceptions are also goals of
treatment. With all activities in this group, involuntary (noncortical)
motor responses are encouraged so that sensory integration may be
achieved (Ayres, 1973).

Drawing and painting group is primarily for the older children who
can express themselves nonverbally on a symbolic level. The drawing
often becomes a catalyst for a discussion of feelings because the
children usually respond to each other's products. The group is
assigned selected themes and encouraged to respond within particular
media. The therapist evaluates the child's response to the media as
well as the content. For example, the task of one drawing group was
to draw a picture of a favorite room at home. In this activity it was
important to note the children's affective response to the task as
well as the content of the drawing. One child depicted his bedroom
and all of his possessions. Another child depicted the kitchen, with
emphasis on the kitchen table and mealtime. With some children, such
a task is so emotionally charged that they deny their real home environment and instead project their dream house.

Puppetry is a fantasy play group for all age children. It
encourages creative thinking and expression of different emotions
through role playing. Psychodramatic play offers a child an opportunity
for reality testing, cognitive stimulation, and socialization. The group
is structured so that each child is allotted a 5-minute period and is
encouraged to tell a story. The audience, which consists of the other
children in the group, is encouraged to participate in the storytelling.

Within the group, issues such as sibling rivalry, competition, limit-setting, individuality, protection, and nurturance are expressed and explored. The interventions made by the therapist encourage storytelling, identify emotions, and make general statements about group issues and responses. The puppet group assists in the differential diagnosis of a child. Psychotic children often become overstimulated and disorganized by such fantasy play and are unable to differentiate reality from fantasy. More often the children's stories become catalysts for each other's play and facilitate the dramatic expression of affect-laden thoughts and conflicts.

E., a 10-year-old child with psycholinguistic difficulty and a history of encopresis, was generally negative and nonverbal, and at times passive aggressive. Through involvement in puppet group, E. was first able to get vicarious pleasure in the other children's play, (particularly where aggressive themes predominated). When he felt less threatened and more comfortable he was able to create his own stories and elaborated on his own aggressive fantasies.

The specific content of each child's story is generally symbolic of his feelings. I., a very guarded child, markedly improved during his hospitalization. His depression lifted and he began to develop his potential. His final puppet play was about a child who broke his ankle, went to the hospital, had a series of tests and treatments, and then went home. His story suggested positive feelings about hospitalization and his discharge.

The focus of the sculpture group is twofold. It is structured to help the older children release aggressive affects in a nonthreatening constructive manner. Clay, plaster, wood work, and metal work are used to facilitate this self-expressive process. The children are encouraged to sublimate and express their feelings through the activity. The sculpture group has been particularly effective with children who have a history of aggressive behavior (fire-setting, fighting, encopresis), withhold these feelings in a structured setting, and explode when their defenses are no longer adequate. The media selected in the sculpture group help the child integrate these feelings. The activity helps channel these feelings and increase the child's awareness of them. With such constructive rechanneling of aggressive impulses the therapist may then explore the motivation and encourage verbalization of the issues.

The sculpture group also helps the children learn to conceptualize forms and spatial relationships three-dimensionally. Collages, puppet construction, mobiles, and stabiles are used to develop such perceptual skills. These goals are implemented once a child is able to release, channel, and repress his feelings appropriately. They demand a higher level of emotional and cognitive functioning. The acts of building, destruction, and creation are used to stimulate ego-development. They are effective media to use with unsocialized aggressive children.

Sensory stimulation group provides an experience wherein the young children have an opportunity to explore and play with a variety of media. Tactile, olfactory, and gustatory stimuli are used to increase the child's awareness of his or her environment. With finger painting, a child can overcome inhibitions, master primitive impulses, and express fantasies. It can facilitate a catharsis of emotional conflicts. M., a 5-year-old, overanxious child, was inhibited affectively and in his play. He was helped to release his underlying rage and become more integrated with finger painting sessions. N., an 8-year-old boy with a history of chronic encopresis, repeatedly made a controlled picture with finger paints and then a messy one. These sessions offered him an opportunity to express and master his conflicts over control within the context of play. In later sessions, he was able to freely enjoy sand play and progress from a sensory/exploratory experience to a higher level fantasy play.

Play group and talking group are two psychotherapy groups. Their emphasis is on encouraging self-expression and peer interaction. Because the stay on the unit is short term, the groups focus on strengthening adaptive functions such as verbalization of feelings, learning self-control, differentiation of thought from action, and learning to be empathic. Although individual dynamics are acknowledged in the context of the group session, the focus is on the group at large and the processes occurring in the here and now. The expectations for each group are contingent on the developmental levels of the children.

The play group is for children functioning on an early latency-age level. It is conducted by the occupational therapist, with a child psychiatry fellow and nurse as co-leaders. Within this group, the children are expected to communicate their feelings via play, games, and activities. The sessions are nondirective and occur within the unit playroom. The therapist encourages the children to translate action into words and make interpretations when indicated (Abramson, Hoffman, and Johns, 1979).

The talking group is for more verbal children in late latency. It is conducted by a child psychiatry fellow and co-led by two nurses. In this group the expectations are similar to adult therapy groups where the patients sit in a circle and discuss their feelings about events on the unit as well as personal issues.

In both the play group and talking group, two general themes predominate. One is separation. The length of hospitalization is short and the children are constantly responding and reacting to the separation from their families as well as to the vicissitudes of the admissions and discharges on the unit. The second major theme centers around the issue of control and caretaking. Many of the children lack internal controls as a result of the tremendous deprivation they have experienced. They crave nurturance from parent-surrogates and may be intensely rivalrous of their peers who are viewed as competitors for the staff's attention. The group experiences foster socialization, requiring control of impulses.

A final group is the weekend evening meeting. This meeting is conducted Sunday evening by the evening nursing staff with the attendance of the doctor "on call" that weekend. At this time the children share with the staff and each other how they spent their weekend, either in the hospital or on pass at home. This meeting is highly structured and its major goal is to help give closure to the child's weekend.

In summary structured groups provide a vehicle for developmental stimulation and psychotherapy for the children on the unit (See Chap. 10 for discussion of Parent-Child Activity Groups).

ACKNOWLEDGMENTS

This chapter was written in consultation with Peter Kaye, Activities Therapist at Mount Sinai Medical Center.

REFERENCES

Abramson, R., Hoffman, L., and Johns, C. (1979). Development and evaluation of a play group for early latency age children on an

inpatient psychiatric unit. *Int. J. Group Psychother.*
Ayres, A.J. (1973). *Sensory Integrations and Learning Disorders.*
   Calif.: Western Psychological Services.
Erikson, E.H. (1977). *Toys and Reason.* New York: Norton.
Freud, A. (1965). *Normality and Pathology in Childhood: Assessment
   of Development.* New York: Int. Univ. Press, pp. 79-84.
Goldenson, R.M., and Hartley, E. (1963). *Children's Play.* New York:
   Crowell.
Greenacre, P. (1971). Discussion of E.A. Galenson. Consideration of
   the nature of thought in childhood play. In *Separation-Individuation:
   Essays in Honor of Margaret S. Mahler.* J.B. McDevitt and C.F.
   Settlage, eds. New York: Int. Univ. Press, pp. 60-69.
Kaplan, F. and Kaplan, T. (1976). *Power of Play.* New York:
   Doubleday/Anchor.
Llorens, L. and Rubin, E. (1967). *Developing Ego Functions in
   Disturbed Children: Occupational Therapy in Milieu.* Detroit:
   Wayne State University.
Lowenfeld, M. (1967). *Play in Childhood.* New York: Science Editions.
Piaget, J. (1962). *Play, Dreams and Imitation in Childhood.* New York:
   Norton Library.
Sarnoff, C. (1976). *Latency.* New York: Aronson.
Schaefer, C. (1976). *The Therapeutic Use of Child's Play.* New York:
   Aronson.
Scheidlinger, S. (1966). The concept of latency: Implications for
   group treatment. *Soc. Casework,* June, pp. 363-367.
Shapiro, T., and Perry, R. (1976). Latency revisited: The age 7
   plus or minus 1. *Psychoanalyt. Study Child 31:* 79-106.
Slavson, S., and Schiffer, M. (1975). *Group Psychotherapies for
   Children.* New York: Int. Univ. Press.
Sutton, B., and Smith, S. (1974). *How to Play with Your Children.*
   New York: Hawthorne.

Chapter 10

PARENT-CHILD ACTIVITY

Elaine Simon

The importance of the parent-child relationship in the child's emotional, cognitive, social, and motor development cannot be over-emphasized. Within the family the child develops ideals, self-esteem, and a unique approach to life tasks. Family members provide the first and most influential models for identification.

Parents who have emotionally disturbed children frequently require training, education, and support. Parent groups, family counseling, and family therapy are all useful modalities (Chilman, 1964). Straughan (1964), for example, allows the parents to observe the therapy of their child through a one-way mirror. Others teach parents behavior modification techniques by methods such as observation, modeling, educational groups, and direct instruction (Hawkins, et al., 1966; Johnson and Brown, 1976; O'Leary and Becker, 1967; Croake and Glover, 1977, and Wahler et al., 1965).

Modeling is a techinque whereby the therapist sets an example to stimulate imitation of behaviors, attitudes, and affects which are more adaptive (Bandura, 1969). This imitation, which is initially rote, becomes internalized with practice. Modeling is effective in changing parental behaviors because learning often is facilitated by observation. Rapid change in the behavior can occur which is then maintained for an extended period of time (Goodman, 1975).

One cannot treat severely disturbed children by simply altering the child's maladaptive behavior pattern. There must be an attempt to modify parental attitudes and/or behaviors that perpetuate the child's symptom picture. For example, parents may be trained to aid the child's development via home educational programs (Gordon, 1969; Morris, 1973; O'Leary and Becker, 1967).

Parents often resist becoming active participants in the child's treatment because they feel as if they are being accused of causing the child's illness. A parent-child activity encourages the parent's active participation without directly focusing on the parental role. An activity is often less threatening to parents and children who lack formal education and find verbal expression taxing. An activity focuses on doing rather than talking. It provides an arena for practice and eliminates the difficult step of translating verbal ideas into actions. The parent(s), the child, sibling(s), and the therapist are all active participants. The activity can be chosen by the therapist or by the

71

family. It can be any activity appropriate for the child's development and of interest to the family: games, painting, puppets, cooking, going for a walk, and so on.

During the activity the interaction between parent and child can be observed:

1. What roles do the various family members assume? Is the parent nurturing, rejecting, authoritarian, passive? Does the child have control over the activity and its outcome?

2. What are the themes and accompanying affects?

3. What methods of communication are utilized by the parent and child? Where do family members choose to sit? Do they work cooperatively? Do they speak to each other? What is the quality of the communication?

4. Are limits set by the parent?

5. Is the child rewarded for appropriate acts?

6. If given a choice, does the family or parent choose an activity appropriate for everyone?

Information about the home life can be gathered; types of play the child prefers, frequency of parent-child interaction, and the quality of this interaction. When the therapist understands the quality of the parent-child interaction, he or she can establish a set of goals. These may be:

1. Change existing roles by helping the parent distinguish between his or her needs and the child's needs. Increase the parent's understanding of the child's behaviors and needs. Help the parent gain confidence with his or her involvement with the child. Help the child respond to parental authority.

2. Increase the frequency of interaction through positive reinforcement such as praise during the activities.

3. Increase appropriate stimulation of the child by educating the parent and suggesting activities. For example, teach the family a board game that they can borrow, encourage imaginative play through a puppet show, or provide sensory stimulation by playing in the sandbox and suggesting a trip to the sand park.

4. Increase and improve communication between the parent and child by pointing out observed behaviors, suggesting changes, or modeling more effective methods of interaction. The choice of activity results in differing amounts and types of communication. For example, the family may need to learn to share limited supplies. Charades improves nonverbal communication skills.

5. Help the parent choose more effective methods of discipline, and model consistent limit-setting.

6. Encourage the parents to acknowledge the child's positive attempts or successes. Provide verbal reinforcement for the parent and child and gradually encourage the parent to spontaneously and regularly

reward the child's positive acts.

7. Carry-over into the home can be fostered by
giving "homework," that is, providing materials
and requesting that the activity be repeated at
home and the project either brought in or discussed.
The parents can borrow appropriate materials or
bring supplies from home.

The major techniques for the therapist during the parent-child
activity are education, choice of appropriate activity, role modeling,
guidance, support and encouragement, and interpretations of maladaptive
interactions.

M., an 8-year-old depressed boy with learning and behavior problems,
was brought to the hospital by his parents because he fought with his
younger brother and misbehaved in school. The family consisted of
the mother, father, and two boys—R., 6 years old, and M. The father
had not been in the home consistently and the mother was illiterate
with many physical ailments. Their marital problems were kept "silent."
M. felt vulnerable and unprotected. He became anxious and depressed,
leading to aggressive behavior which the mother was incapable of
controlling.

One of the first goals of the weekly sessions attended by the
mother and two children was to instill leadership in the mother. The
activity chosen was cooking, something she did well. The therapist
modeled taking leadership when it became evident that the mother
couldn't assume this role. Leadership meant being the organizer, giving
each member of the family a job, and being "boss."

The next week the mother was "boss" (a term that became popular
with the family). Behaviors were interpreted: For example, "M. is
not doing the job you asked him to do, I wonder why?" Both the mother
and children changed. She began to take responsibility for the
children and the children, especially M., were relieved and were able
to accept limits. M.'s behavior improved.

A second family included a mother and two boys, J., 8 years old
and F., 11. They were referred from a medical clinic because the
mother seemed incapable of controlling the children.

J. had a symbiotic relationship with his mother. In school he was
electively mute, aggressive, and had difficulty following rules, waiting
his turn, completing tasks, and playing with other children. The
home situation was marked by a great deal of sibling rivalry and fighting.
The older boy, F., named after the father who had not lived with the
family for several years, reminded the mother of her ex-husband. F.,
enuretic, hyperactive and phobic, felt rejected by the mother, whereas
the mother and J. shared a bed, excluding F. because of his enuresis.

The mother was gently instructed that each member of the family
have a separate bed. Family meetings focused on problems in school
and at home. Often, the mother would act in a rejecting fashion toward
F. who would lash out at J., provoking a fight. J. would have a
temper tantrum, preventing further discussion. The staff decided that
a parent-child activity would provide a structured positive experience
for everyone.

A series of graded activities were planned. Initially, each family
member was provided with his or her own supplies and each would
complete his or her own product (parallel level of interaction). The
next step required that the supplies be shared and the final step that
the mother and children not only share supplies but work together on
a group project such as a mural. The therapist participated, observed

interactions, made interventions, and provided materials for homework assignment. Each week, the family was asked to repeat the project at home and to bring in the products. J. had difficulty completing the projects during the session but would complete them at home. Mother and F. began to interact with a positive attitude during the activities. The quality of the family's interactions and communication improved even though the mother had a great deal of difficulty noting the children's attempts and successes. She would become very involved in her own work, need approval from the therapist, and would seemingly forget the children. She received much reassurance and began to provide some acknowledgment and praise for the children.

A parent-child activity is a treatment modality distinct from other methods such as family therapy, family counseling, or parent education. It is primarily a directive therapy whereby the therapist chooses appropriate activities and actively participates along with the family members. This allows for the evaluation of the parent-child relationship. Activities are chosen in order to promote increased communication and understanding among the family members, clearer definition of parental roles, more effective discipline methods, and/or provide stimulation for the child's continued development. The activities are graded developmentally from one session to the next while products provide concrete evidence of change. Carry-over into the home is encouraged by giving homework, sharing of supplies, and discussion of the play interactions at home. In the second case illustration, more positive communication and interactions between the mother and children were achieved and there was a carry-over into the home. In the first illustration, the mother was able to change, becoming more of a mother. This led to a decrease in the child's symptoms and an improvement in his functioning.

REFERENCES

Bandura, A. (1969). *Principles of Behavior Modification*. New York: Holt, Rinehart, and Winston.

Chilman, C. (1964). The crisis and challenge of low income families in the 1960's: Implications for parent education. *J. Marr. Fam.* 26: 39-43.

Croake, J., and Glover, K. (1977). A history and evaluation of parent education. *Fam. Coord.* 26: 151-158.

Goodman, E.O. (1975). Modeling, a method of parent education. *Fam. Coord.* 24: 7-11.

Gordon, I.J. (1969). Stimulation via parent education. *Children* 16: 57.

Hawkins, R., Peterson, R., Schweid, E., and Bijou, S. (1966). Behavior therapy in the home: Amelioration of problem parent-child relations with parent in a therapeutic role. *J. Exp. Child Psychol.* 4: 99-107.

Johnson, S., and Brown, R. (1976). Producing behavior change in parents. In *The Therapeutic Use of Child's Play*. C. Schaefer, ed. New York: Aronson, pp. 637-653.

Morris, A. (1973). Parent education being carried out in a pediatric clinic. *Clin. Pediat.* 12: 235-239.

O'Leary, K., O'Leary, S., and Becker, W. (1967). Modification of deviant sibling interaction in the home. *Behav. Res. Ther.* 5: 113-120.

Straughan, J. (1964). Treatment with child and mother in the playroom. *Behav. Res. Ther.* 2: 37-41.

Wahler, R., Wienkel, G., Peterson, R., and Morrison, D. (1965). Mothers as behavior therapists for their own children. *Behav. Res. Ther.* 3: 113-124.

Chapter 11

AN EDUCATIONAL PROGRAM FOR THE HOSPITALIZED, EMOTIONALLY DISTURBED CHILD

Norman A. Friedman

To the latency-age child, school is equivalent to the work world of the adult. An average of 6 hours per day of school becomes the focal point of his or her life. In school, the child develops his academic skills, forms peer group relationships, finds new models for identification, and learns to relate to various authority figures. Children who require psychiatric hospitalization usually are unable to function in their school setting.

Most children on the inpatient and day patient unit at Mount Sinai Medical Center come from the nearby community, which consists of low socioeconomic minority groups. It is therefore not surprising that the average pupil is 2 years behind grade level in reading, comprehension, and other academic skills. Many are advanced in the local schools up to the third grade. At age 9, they may be nonreaders with little knowledge of basic phonics. Even those students from more favorable environments with higher I.Q. ranges usually do not perform at grade level because of their psychopathology. With few exceptions, the average student in the hospital school requires a great deal of individual programming, remedial and tutorial work, and constant positive reinforcement within a warm supportive atmosphere.

The hospital school experience is a rewarding and accepting learning situation. A youngster from a culturally deprived home with severe symptomatology cannot function in a class of 30 or more children taught by a harassed teacher with minimum, if any, special education preparation. In a setting of five to eight in a class, such youngsters can start to learn and begin to overcome educational lags and deficits.

In a psychiatric hospital setting, the school plays a number of different roles. It is an educational facility, a diagnostic tool for learning disabilities, a social evaluator for individual and group behavior, and a guidance and disposition reference for each child.

The smallness of the site at Mount Sinai does not permit a specific elementary class for each grade. There are two classes for the inpatient unit and one for the day treatment program. The work range within a given level is individualized sufficiently to cover a latitude of at least 3 academic years. This requires a great deal of preparation by the teacher because the children need individual attention and work assignments.

Within the first week of schooling, each child is evaluated in an after-school tutorial program. Reading, comprehension, and arithmetic disabilities are accurately pinpointed and individualized remedial programs established. The tutorial work is coordinated with actual class assignments as well as with the remediation provided by the occupational therapist and other unit personnel.

Positive reinforcement is constantly used as an ego-building technique. It is not unusual for students to be proudly sent to the principal's office for recognition of a 100 percent paper or the mastery of a new skill. Commendation cards are frequently given. The children display them on the unit, and show them to the staff and to their parents. To further enrich the curriculum, departmental programs are scheduled in the areas of health, education, music, crafts, and recreation. At times, educational trips, for example, to museums, are arranged. A varied audiovisual section is employed in order to help bridge wide gaps in the fund of knowledge of culturally deprived youngsters.

Aggressive and provocative behavior occurs periodically. Firm limits are set and the child is made aware that behavior is accepted only within the set tolerance of the structure. Conduct disruptive to the group is not condoned. The unruly child is asked to take a time-out outside the class with the admonition that at this time he or she is not able to accept the school setting, but can return as soon as he or she feels in control of his or her actions. A quiet period in the school corridor alcove with a nurse or attendant usually provides sufficient reconstitution within a short period of time. When the child asks to reenter the class, he or she does so with a minimum of attention.

During the course of a school year a small number of children under 5 years of age are admitted to the hospital. Since the educational program is geared to school-age children who function on at least a reading readiness level and who have the ability to function in a peer group of close to first grade, the inpatient school cannot adequately service the under-5 population. Such children attend a neighborhood therapeutic nursery school which is able to provide an educational program for the very young child. This program consists of half-day classes. Some of these children can attend the inpatient school for the other half day, particularly for the visual arts program.

Autistic and extremely regressed organic youngsters seldom can tolerate a full school day in a class not geared entirely to their needs. Special time sequences are established based on their specific needs. Every child, however, attends school. This is regarded as a necessary part of the treatment program, even if it is limited.

Prior to discharge, the child is prepared for his new school adjustment. The guidance department or school administration of the receiving facility is contacted and a description of the child's functioning and accomplishments in the hospital school setting is shared. Recommendations are made for new class placements, work levels, and peer group assignments that will keep frustration and adjustment at optimal levels.

Some students are not residential treatment candidates nor, at the time of discharge, are they able to function in a normal school environment. The need to provide a meaningful service for such children resulted in the formation of a day school treatment program. Many youngsters can return home and be seen on an outpatient basis, but cannot cope with an immediate public school placement. When such students continue in a day hospital school program for a minimum of 6 months to 1 year, they can make the readjustment to home and regular school at a slower and more acceptable pace. Day school classes help bridge the gap between full-time residence and home and regular school attendance. Problems can be dealt with before they become acute because of the intensive daily contact. If need be, short rehospitalization is arranged until a conflict is resolved. The day program also allows for continued parent involvement. Proper use of day classes provides latitude in the school reassignment of pupils. For example, a child does not have to return to a facility during the middle of a term or during a very stressful period such as exam week. A more logical calendar can be utilized for the student's best interests, thus helping him or her make a more therapeutic transition to the community school.

The teacher chosen to work in a psychiatric hospital school must present a personality profile far beyond what is expected of a pedagogue of normal children. Basic qualifications and certification in special education are simply not enough. The pathology of the students makes it essential that the teacher be flexible and spontaneous in his or her approach to teaching and pupil management. The mood swings of one pupil in the class can cause a contagious reaction which can only be dealt with a quick shift of direction and plans. Emotionally disturbed children are very needy and constantly test authority figures. The teacher needs great ingenuity, humor, poise, and the ability to withstand high frustration. An excellently prepared lesson can be easily shattered. It is a repeatedly giving situation, often with little results or gratifications that one can measure by the standard yardstick. The teacher must be able to maintain control of the class at all times, without appearing punitive or rejecting. He or she must provide each child instruction in a variety of subjects according to ability and grade level.

As a close, warm, and nonthreatening authority figure, the teacher is often the recipient of much transferential material from the student. These highlights plus the academic progress have to be shared with other team members for better understanding and more effective treatment planning. Children may exhibit quite different symptoms and behaviors in school, on the unit, in groups, in psychotherapy, and so on.

One detailed report is described:

J., a 10-year-old neighborhood youngster, was admitted to the unit with serious problems of hyperactivity, fighting, and refusal to do work in school. His school was forced to suspend him from his fifth grade class because of the severity of the symptoms. The home was chaotic and disorganized. J.'s father was in and out of the house, his mother was depressed, and two younger siblings were beginning to have school problems.

Upon entering class, J. was quiet and controlled but extremely negative and hostile. He complained that he should not be here and that he would not do what he did in his former school so we "would also throw him out." Even though he was reassured that the staff understands his problems and would not reject him, he turned over a desk in the room and disrupted the class. This was followed by curses, running about, and scattering other pupils' work. The teacher restrained him, removed him from the room, and with an arm around him in a friendly and protective manner quietly explained that at this moment he was not ready to be in class, that he would be welcome to return as soon as he felt in sufficient control.

After sitting with a nurse in the hallway, J. created another disturbance. He was taken down to the ward which he found empty of companionship. J. asked to return to class for the afternoon session. With slight hesitation he entered the room. He was greeted by the teacher in the same manner as the other students, with no mention made of the morning episode. J. was assigned to his regular work which he completed poorly, but without incident. Despite his grade placement in the fifth grade, J. was reading on an 1.8 level with extremely poor comprehension and limited vocabulary. As he began to trust his tutor, J. confided his fears and embarrassment due to his limited academic abilities.

The speech and hearing therapist discovered that J. had significant auditory perceptual problems, whereas his visual perceptual functions were fairly good. Verbal commands were thus given in a short direct fashion. He was tutored to sight-read words rather than use phonics.

As time progressed, J.'s frustration tolerance increased and he accepted the structure of the school. He was well motivated. All progress was noted and positively reinforced. Commendation cards were issued, good work was displayed on the class progress board, and he was rewarded by being given special privileges. With the absence of home and school pressures, J. was able to develop greater control over his aggressive outbursts when provoked by stress or anxiety. He became well liked within his peer group and his scholastic advancement, although limited, added greatly to his self-esteem. At the end of his 3-month stay his reading had advanced to a 3.2 level, a more acceptable attainment for his actual grade placement.

After discharge, he was placed in the day school program where he and his mother continued to receive support. He did not have to return to school in the middle of the term and both J. and his mother had several months of intensive treatment. He completed the full school term in the day program while arrangements were made with his former school's guidance department for a smooth transition back to that school.

The success of a hospital school program is very difficult to measure due to the multiplicity of variables. It is of prime importance that the school program be fully integrated into the treatment plans of the child. The teaching of severely disturbed children requires that the teacher be able to assess the child's academic level, understand the intrapsychic and interpersonal conflicts which interfere with the child's performance, and understand how neuropsychological deficits can prevent adequate learning. At the same time, other staff members have to be aware of how school can be both anxiety-provoking as well as rewarding to the child. A key to success with the child is to find his strengths and help him compensate for his deficits.

SUGGESTED READINGS

Berkowitz, P.H., and Rothman, E. (1967). Public education for
    disturbed children in New York City. New York: Thomas.
Cruickshank, W. (1971). *Psychology of Exceptional Children and
    Youths.* Englewood Cliffs, N.J.: Prentice-Hall.
Grossman, H. (1965). *Teaching the Emotionally Disturbed.* New York:
    Holt, Rinehart, and Winston.
Hewett, F.N. (1968). *The Emotionally Disturbed Child in the Classroom.*
    New York: Allyn and Bacon.

Chapter 12

PRIMARY NURSING IN CHILD PSYCHIATRY

Mary Rehill

Children who require inpatient psychiatric or residential treatment
are children who cannot be assessed or treated adequately on an
outpatient basis. Their evaluation and treatment in the hospital or
residential center extends over the 24-hour day and not simply during
the time the child participates in psychotherapy and group therapy.
The nursing staff plays the key role in the milieu assessment and
treatment of these children because they have the ongoing 24-hour
responsibility for overall patient care. Unlike other staff members,
the nursing staff participates in virtually all aspects of the diagnostic
and treatment process. A nurse is available to the child at any time of the
day or night. The nurse helps the child in his or her daily living
experiences (grooming, meals, baths), participates in the various
structured activities, escorts the child throughout the hospital for
consultations and diagnostic tests, and interacts with the child during
free time. The nurse observes the child's behavior, nature of interactions with adults and peers, and level of involvement in a variety of
situations. The nurse tries to understand and respond to the child's
"needs of care and nurturance" (Fagin, 1974).

The strengthening of the milieu program at the Mount Sinai Medical
Center Child Psychiatry Unit has been accompanied by increased
staffing in nursing and therapeutic activities and a reorganization of
the Department of Nursing. This has enabled the nurse to enhance
his or her role as an effective contributor to the interdisciplinary
psychiatric team. In 1976, the Department of Nursing decentralized
leadership positions, emphasizing unit-based management. Previously,
the child psychiatry unit was managed by a head nurse and an assistant
head nurse under the leadership of assistant supervisors who were
centrally based within the Department of Psychiatry, sharing the 24-hour
responsibility of four adult units and the Child Psychiatry Inpatient
Unit. Their duties limited their contact with individual units and
consequently nursing practice was inhibited by the lack of supervision
available. The reorganization created the position of a clinical supervisor who has 24-hour responsibility and accountability for patient care
on the unit.

Approximately 20 nursing staff members are required in order to
adequately staff all shifts on a 24-hour, 7-day-a-week basis. A staff/
patient ratio of 1:3 to 4 enables the nursing staff to practice primary

nursing. The primary nurse's first task involves developing a relationship with the child. It is only within the context of such a relationship
that the nurse, as well as any other staff member, can help the child
"increase adaptive behavior and decrease maladaptive behavior" (Wardle,
1974, p. 89). In conjunction with the other team members, the primary
nurse coordinates the 24-hour therapeutic care for the individual child.

At the time of the intake interview, the family visits the unit and
receives a preadmission information list which recommends clothing, food,
and toys to bring to the hospital and explains visiting and phone call
policies. The family's questions about procedures are answered and
their anxiety alleviated to facilitate adjustment to the unit. The nursing
staff member who participates in the intake process usually becomes the
primary nurse for that child. On the day of admission, the family is
escorted to unit by this nurse who conducts the admission interview
together with the primary therapist. Occasionally, staffing patterns
may interfere and the primary nurse assigned at intake may not be
available. In that case, the family is then informed of the name of
the nurse who will be with them on the day of admission.

The preparation for admission has proven to be invaluable in the
adjustment phase of hospitalization. It is much less traumatic for the
child and family to be separated from each other when they have
previously visited the unit and met the staff. The primary nurse and
the primary therapist support the child and family during the difficult
separation time. In contrast, "emergency" admissions (patients who
have not been evaluated via the formal intake process) have little or
no preparation for hospitalization and may need to be physically separated
from the family. The treatment goal of the first few days is to undo
this trauma so that a trusting relationship may become established.

The activities of daily living (ADL) are clearly outlined for the
children. They know when to make their beds, brush their teeth,
bathe, dress, eat, go to bed, and so on. The nursing staff monitors
the child's responses to the expected behaviors in order to develop a
rational diagnostic and therapeutic plan. For example, a child who
cannot tie his or her shoelaces can have a lesson in tying. If the child
cannot learn from direction, one needs to pinpoint the cause. Such a
child may have a receptive language impairment, a motor problem, or
an impairment of his intelligence. There may be an emotional component
such as negativism. During the interdisciplinary staff conferences the
observations from the various disciplines are integrated in order to
come to a comprehensive diagnosis.

Children in residential settings frequently attempt to play one staff
member against the other. For example, the children are expected to
bathe at least every other night. They may tell the evening staff that
they have taken a bath in the morning and that the day staff did not
communicate this information. In this way the children try to arrange
a repetition of the parental conflicts at home. Unless there is adequate
communication, the staff cannot make appropriate interventions.

During unstructured activity time (more commonly known as free
time) there is a relaxation of the routine in order that the children have
the opportunity for self-expression, allowing them to demonstrate their
capabilities or liabilities. The nurse observes the types of activities a
child selects, for example, ball games and table games, and how the
child chooses peers or adults for interactions. The nurse assesses the
child's ability or inability to initiate an activity independently and
whether the child's functioning is developmentally appropriate, regressed,
or advanced.

Unstructured time promotes individual expression and allows the development of spontaneous groups by the children (Sheimo, Paynter, and Szurek, 1949). Their underlying concerns can be inferred by observing the activities they select, the qualities of interactions, and the noise level on the unit. For example, when the children are very anxious they may become more aggressive and the unit becomes louder. It is crucial for the staff to try to understand dynamically the causes of the increased anxiety. When the children feel unprotected they may "test limits," play cops and robbers games, make paper guns, and be more aggressive with each other and/or with the staff. The staff needs to determine the origin of the children's feelings. For example, staff vacations, staff resignations, changes in staff assignments, intrastaff conflicts, or an inability to control a psychotic or aggressive child may make the children anxious, feel unprotected, and lead to disruptive behavior on the unit.

Structured treatment programs are invaluable. However, a comprehensive program for emotionally disturbed children which meets the needs of the individual child requires staff who can be flexible (Whittaker, 1975). Children experience free time differently from structured time. For example, a child with impaired ego boundaries cannot tolerate free time. "Borderline" children may function very well in structured activities such as school and activities groups. In one-to-one situations such children may perform quite well. However, during free time they manifest their severe anxiety by provoking staff and other children. It is important to allow the free time in order to effectively assess the children's pathology.

The nursing staff supervision of free time promotes the development of a variety of relationships. Understanding and acceptance of the child by the nurse fosters a trusting relationship. A child may become attached to a particular staff member or members other than the primary nurse. He or she supports the child's selection and attempts to understand the reasons for the development of the particular relationships. The child's dynamics can be elucidated and a rational overall treatment approach developed.

In contrast to members of other disciplines whose responsibilities on the unit may be more limited, the nursing staff's role and functions allow for a greater degree of flexibility in response to the children's needs. Nurses are present when issues arise on the unit. The nurse is able to provide immediate intervention and on-the-spot ego interpretation or ego support (Noshpitz, 1962). The nurse provides support and understanding to help the child understand him or herself and make the effort to improve.

Most difficulties revolve around interpersonal issues. The nurse needs not only to stop a fight between the children but also to understand the underlying cause, help the children resolve conflicts with better control, and relate the child's difficulty in the hospital to the problems at home. When the nurse senses that the child is attempting to provoke a fight, he or she can explore the connections to the conflicts between the child and the parents.

The nursing staff members are available to the family throughout the entire hospitalization. The parents are encouraged to discuss their child's progress with the nursing staff during visiting hours or by telephone. The parents recognize the nurse as the person who is involved daily with their child.

Not infrequently, competitive conflicts may arise between the parents and the nursing staff. The parents may view the nurse as a competitor for the parental role and may project their guilt onto them. The parents may provoke arguments and accuse the nurse of maltreating their child.

On the other hand, the nurse, observing the obvious inadequacies of the parents, may consciously or unconsciously attempt to "rescue" the child from the pathogenic family. The nurse needs to remain as objective as possible in order to help decrease the parent's guilt so that they can allow the staff to effectively treat the child.

The nurse serves a very important function as a co-therapist in family sessions. He or she can help the child express him or herself in order to begin to resolve the conflicts within the family unit. This support of the child occurs while empathizing with the parent's needs.

A nurse functions as a co-leader of the parents group. In this meeting, there are many discussions of specific issues relating to the care of the children. The nurse can provide factual information, while at the same time helping the parents deal with their own separation problems from the child.

Thus, the nursing staff, along with the other staff, begin to understand the family dynamics and the transferential meaning of the parents' reactions to the nurse. The nurse tries to remain objective, avoid conflict and competition, and encourages the parent to become a collaborator in the treatment of the child rather than an antagonist.

Many of the children hospitalized on the unit lack adequate internal controls. They become easily frustrated and may provoke or be provoked into fighting. The staff has to provide external controls by setting limits on inappropriate and dangerous behavior. These controls are provided in a variety of ways. The most common are verbal interventions. The staff may simply redirect the child away from a potentially explosive situation; the staff may be able to discuss with the child his or her lack of control, or the staff may understand the meaning of the child's behavior and communicate this to the child. Such an ego interpretation may successfully stop the inappropriate behavior.

If verbal interventions are not successful, a time-out away from the area of conflict can be very effective. At times, physical controls such as holding the child, or brief isolation from the group for severely agitated behavior may be necessary. At other times psychotropic medication may be required to control the child's anxiety, hyperactivity, and impulsivity.

Since the nursing staff has the 24-hour responsibility for the care of the children, the nurses and nursing assistants are the ones who usually provide limit-setting for the children. Blau and Slaff (1964) emphasized the role of the nurse as mother-surrogate for the children. No mention was made of the role of male nursing staff members.

Social roles as well as physiological differences may limit the experience women have had in dealing with and controlling aggressive behavior. Aggressive children, especially boys, look toward the male members of the staff as models for identification and as auxiliary egos who can provide external controls by effective limit-setting. Female nursing staff members as well as other staff may feel uncomfortable dealing with potentially aggressive behavior. This usually occurs when the staff member is new to the unit. The children perceive that staff's anxiety and can react by "testing limits" with that particular staff member(s) as a way of trying to master the anxiety of not being able to be controlled.

The children feel more comfortable when they know that the staff who take care of them are in control. If the males on the unit (the male nursing assistants and male nurses) are recognized by the staff and patients as the only ones who can effectively set limits on the children's behavior, problems occur if there are no male nursing staff on duty on a particular day. The female staff on duty may become anxious about controlling aggressive behavior; the children perceive this anxiety, become more anxious themselves, and defensively become more aggressive. Most nursing staff master these feelings of anxiety and acquire the skills needed to limit inappropriate and potentially aggressive behavior. The children, of course, perceive the staff's greater comfort with limit-setting and in turn respond to verbal interventions more readily, reducing the need for physical control.

Some staff mistake the use of limit-setting as a punitive measure. It is crucial for all staff members to realize that children with fragile ego structures and poor impulse control require external limits until they can begin to acquire internal limits. The therapeutic program can only be effective when both the children and staff feel there is a reasonable control of asocial impulses. Limit-setting, done in a nonpunitive manner, is an essential ingredient in the therapeutic process.

At times, staff conflicts arise over the role of the limit-setter in the overall treatment plan. For example, when a child becomes disruptive in an aspect of the program where the nursing staff is usually not involved, a nursing staff member may be called to help control the child or the child may be returned to the unit. Nursing staff members (or child care workers in residential treatment centers) may view themselves and be viewed by others simply as "policemen." This, of course, overlooks the importance of limit-setting as an essential ingredient in the treatment of aggressive children. On the other hand, other staff members may view limit-setting as outside their purview. For example, a primary therapist may feel that he or she should not be the one to set limits with the child because it would "interfere" with the therapy; psychotherapeutic treatment of aggressive children with severe ego deficits includes providing external controls. Exercising these controls promotes rather than interferes with the developing psychotherapeutic relationship. In the treatment of severely disturbed aggressive children there cannot be a psychotherapist-administrator split (Harrison, McDermott, and Chethik, 1969).

As with the other treatment plans, the problem of limit-setting requires an interdisciplinary approach. Staff members have to develop an understanding of the specificity of each other's role as well as the overlapping of certain functions. The nursing staff members are the ones with the greatest expertise in limit-setting, yet other staff members need to share in this function when they interact with the children.

The nursing staff coordinates the activities of supportive services from the general hospital to the unit. Since one aim of the unit is to attempt to create a noninstitutional atmosphere, special considerations are required from these services.

The Dietary Department makes every attempt to accommodate the unit. Meals are served family style, with each child having an assigned seat at one of four tables. Some of the staff eat with the children and the children help set up, serve, and clean up on a rotational basis. Meals are selected by the nursing staff from a pediatric menu in order to coordinate the likes and dislikes of the everchanging population. There are barbecues, picnics in the park, lunches for special trips, special occasion party cakes (birthday), and holiday specialties (turkey to be carved on Thanksgiving and Christmas). The dieticians are available; they make daily rounds, counsel and teach the staff and children, and are particularly helpful in formulating treatment plans for children with special dietary needs, for example, those who are diabetic, obese, and malnourished. At times the dietician participates in the community meeting.

The Building Service (Housekeeping) staff have demonstrated under-

standing of the behaviors of disturbed children. The regular staff
consider themselves and are considered by the staff and children as part
of the unit staff. They are familiar with the patients and, at times,
with the families who are from the local community. They often serve
as interpreters for the non-Spanish-speaking staff. Their important
role for the children may be recognized in that two veteran housekeeping
staff members are called "Mama" and "Poppy" by all patients and staff
on the unit.

There are a host of people from the institution who have demonstrated
unique responses to the children. It is not unusual for a patient to
develop a relationship with someone from outside the designated treatment team. These interactions are then monitored by the nursing staff.

In summary, the multifaceted role of the nurse on the child
psychiatry unit is fostered by the variety of interactions between
nurses, patients, and other staff members.

REFERENCES

Blau, A., and Slaff, B. (1964). Child psychiatry division in a general
    hospital. *N.Y. State J. Med. 64:* 1096-1100.
Fagin, C.M. (1974). *Readings in Child and Adolescent Psychiatric
    Nursing.* St. Louis: Mosby.
Harrison, S., McDermott, J., and Chethik, M. (1969). Residential
    treatment of children: The psychotherapist-administrator. *J. Am.
    Acad. Child Psychiatry 8:* 385-410.
Noshpitz, J. (1962). Notes on the theory of residential treatment.
    J. Am. Acad. Child Psychiatry 1: 284-296.
Sheimo, S.L., Paynter, J., and Szurek, S.A. (1949). Staff problems
    with a spontaneous patient group. In *Inpatient Care for the
    Psychotic Child.* S.A. Szurek, I.N. Berlin, and M.J. Boatman, eds.
    Palo Alto, Calif.: Science and Behavior Books, 1971, pp. 122-137.
Wardle, C.J. (1974). Residential care of child with conduct disorders.
    In *The Residential Psychiatric Treatment of Children.* P. Barker,
    ed. New York: Halstead Press.
Whittaker, J. (1975). The ecology of child treatment: A developmental/
    educational approach to the therapeutic milieu. *J. Aut. Childh.
    Schiz. 5:* 223-237.

Chapter 13

THE USE OF PSYCHOTROPIC MEDICATION WITHIN AN INPATIENT MILIEU FOR CHILDREN

Arnold Cohen

During the past decade there have been innumerable studies dealing with the use of psychotropic medication in childhood psychiatric disorders. The classification of medication, the clinical pharmacology, the clinical effects, and the underlying central nervous system effects of the psychotropic agents are discussed in the literature, for example, Weiner (1977). White (1977) discusses the specific psychopharmacological agents, side effects, adverse effects, clinical indications, and dosage range for medications that have been used for controlling psychiatric symptoms in childhood.

This chapter discusses the attitudes and use of medication on an inpatient child psychiatry service: How a clinical decision is arrived at to either use or not use medication in the treatment of the children.

A limited number of medications have been selected for use on the inpatient unit at Mount Sinai Medical Center so that the staff becomes familiar with the therapeutic ranges, therapeutic effects, as well as side effects of the drugs. Chlorpromazine, trifluoroperazine, and occasionally haloperidol are three major tranquilizers that are considered when the target symptoms are severe agitation, psychotic anxiety, hallucinations, delusions, or other signs of thought disorder. Chlorpromazine and haloperidol are also used with children who have severe uncontrollable aggressive or tantrum behavior. Chlorpromazine is most useful where some sedation would be therapeutic. Trifluoroperazine is used more frequently when psychotic withdrawal is present and when sedation should be avoided. Haloperidol is particularly helpful when agitation and unprovoked aggression are serious problems unresponsive to other medications.

Imipramine is used as an antidepressant, at times to control enuresis, and occasionally to treat hyperkinesis. Methylphenidate is the most frequently used stimulant and diphenhydramine is a good safe nighttime sedative which can also control hyperactivity in young children. Diphenhydramine can also control psychotic anxiety in children who cannot tolerate major tranquilizers.

The major problem that confronts the treatment team is not which medication to use for the particular target symptom, but rather whether medication should be used in a particular clinical circumstance, or whether it should be avoided. In general, a child and his symptoms must be reviewed from the criteria of intrapsychic forces, external environmental realities, biological vulnerabilities, and the progress (or lack of progress) of normal development. The effect of medication on development must always be considered. Medications control symptoms but do not alter internal dynamics and may prevent a child from being able to express his inner state to the outside world. The therapeutic effects may be state dependent. On the other hand, medication may positively alter the response of a child's external environment to the child.

Children enter the inpatient psychiatric service with a wide range of problems. These problems run the gamut from psychotic disorders, to conduct disturbances, attention problems, acute and chronic anxiety, and related neurotic and borderline character disorders. The issue that distinguishes most of these children from the general childhood psychiatric population is not the nature of the disorder, but the fact that they cannot function or be maintained in their natural community.

When a child is first admitted to the unit the staff helps the child become comfortable while concomitantly beginning the evaluation process. The diagnostic assessment includes a clinical symptomatic diagnostic statement, which includes the relative contributions of development, biological vulnerability, environmental, and intrapsychic forces. Children are not usually given behavior-altering medication during the first days of hospitalization so that these factors can be clearly evaluated. A medication-free period permits an assessment of the effect of separation from home upon a child's symptoms and gives an indication of how a stable, consistent environment can positively affect behavior. After a child's response to hospitalization is assessed, the nature of his or her symptoms defined, and a baseline level of functioning in the therapeutic milieu ascertained, one then can consider the role of medication.

In the history of the Mount Sinai Medical Center Child Psychiatry Inpatient Unit, medication has been in and out of favor at different times. This has been due in part to a desire to reconcile the belief, on the one hand, that the child's symptoms are but a necessary expression of a child's inner experience and the belief, on the other hand, that suffering deserve relief. If one relieves the suffering, one may inhibit one's ability to understand and help the child to master his conflict. If one conceptualizes symptomatic behavior simply in psychodynamic terms to the exclusion of other points of views, one accepts the challenge of helping the child to master his conflicts mainly with psychotherapeutic modalities.

A child's severe unrelenting symptoms can be frustrating to his or her caretakers. Mental health professionals are sometimes overwhelmed by their impotence in the face of florid pathology. Medication allows the staff member to be active and feel in control rather than feel passive and helpless. In fact, a child may seem much "better" while on medication.

The decision-making process as to whether or not to give medication sometimes leads to conflict among the staff. Some feel that a child's suffering should be alleviated by medication, whereas others feel that he or she should be helped with psychotherapeutic and/or behavioral techniques. For example, members of the nursing staff, who are with the child 24 hours a day and view the severity of the symptoms and their interference in daily functioning, may feel a child should be on medication. On the other hand, the primary therapist and his or her supervisor (attending child psychiatrist), who view the symptoms psycho-dynamically, may feel that the child should be treated without medication but with verbal and behavioral techniques. At times, a dramatic confrontation over "medication" may erupt. This may often be symptomatic of an underlying staff conflict which takes the form of an ideological conflict over the use of medication. Over time, with greater education and more open communication channels among all staff members, a confluent view has prevailed. For example, a child's inner experience is difficult to reach if anxiety or other symptoms overwhelm the child. Rarely does medication make a child so symptom-free that his or her symptoms become unavailable for scrutiny.

Extreme aggression or serious psychotic symptomatology often prevents a full assessment of the child and his or family. Such behavior is quite disorganizing to the other children and it disrupts attempts to provide an even and consistent milieu. Therefore, some children receive major tranquilizers early during their hospital stay. A child with episodic outbursts of aggression at first may receive the medication on a *pro re nata* (p.r.n.) basis, whereas a psychotic child will be given a standing dose of medication.

The large majority of the children who do receive medication receive it after the initial evaluation period and after discussion by all the staff. Because a child's stay in the hospital is fairly brief, the staff needs to consider early during the hospital course whether the child has target symptoms that are medication-responsive. A trial of medication may be offered unless it is clear that the child's symptoms subside or are controllable on the general milieu. A child who improves simply with the structure of the hospital certainly does not need medication.

Parents may be frightened about the administration of medication to their child. Their anxiety may be engendered by adverse publicity in the media or by their guilt and fears that their child is very sick. Many parents who are or were or who have relatives who were or are addicted to drugs are often frightened that the medication may become addictive. It is crucial that the staff discuss the use of medication with the parents and child prior to its administration.

Medications are generally administered in small doses and carefully titrated. Behavioral responses and side effects are monitored. The clinical effects are discussed in conferences and appropriate changes in type and dosage are implemented.

Medications suppress symptoms; they do not cure them. Environmental change, behavioral modification, individual and group therapy, psychoeducational techniques, and a whole host of other interventions may be of much greater long-term value to the child. Yet, a less severely symptomatic child is more engageable, can interact more appropriately with the other children, be more successful in school, and be less likely to begin a chain reaction of disorganized behavior. Nonpsychotic, conduct-disturbed children who are easily involved in group contagious reactions, receive p.r.n. medication when the ward is in an unstable state in contrast to psychotic and anxious children who, when they receive p.r.n. medication, do so when the unit is in a more stable state (Hoffman and Bertinelli, 1981).

If a child can remain in the hospital for a long period of time, the medication may be decreased because other treatments have more long-term benefit on intrapsychic processes and cognitive development. Towards the end of hospitalization, symptom flare-ups do occur and medication may then have to be increased.

Medication is never offered as the major therapeutic modality. Medication, whether it be a major tranquilizer, antidepressant, or stimulant, never cures the core of the problem, but there are certainly many situations in which it can be extremely useful. In the presence of a supportive or workable family system, some children can be returned home on maintenance medication. The decrease in the child's behavioral problems may allow for more appropriate, giving, and consistent relationships with his or her parents, teachers, and friends. If a child must be referred for residential placement, the experience with medication in the hospital can be transmitted to the placement agency. Some children cannot be placed in a residential treatment center because of the severity of their symptoms. Medication, along with the rest of the treatment, may decrease the child's symptoms sufficiently so that they can be accepted by a community or a residential facility.

REFERENCES

Hoffman, L., and Bertinelli, A. (1981). Use of PRN medication on an inpatient child psychiatry unit. Manuscript in preparation.
Weiner, J., ed. (1977). *Psychopharmacology in Childhood and Adolescence.* New York: Basic Books.
White, J. (1977). *Pediatric Pharmacology: A Practical Guide.* Baltimore: Willaims & Wilkins.

Chapter 14

POSTHOSPITAL TREATMENT

Lois Shein

Posthospital care is a most important phase in the treatment process of the hospitalized child. Long before he or she is ready to leave the hospital, disposition plans must be thought through, arrived at, and if possible, finalized in order to ensure that the therapeutic effects of hospitalization are not interrupted.

The parents' wishes play a great role in determining the optimal recommendation given for the child. They must be involved in the decision-making process and understand the rationale for the particular posthospital plan. They are the ones who have the responsibility to make decisions regarding *their* child. These decisions are often fraught with a myriad of complex and conflicting emotions. When the staff can recognize the conflicts they can assist the parents in their decision-making. What happens to the child after discharge determines the long-range success of hospitalization (Whittaker, 1975).

In a short-term hospital facility the staff must consider the question of disposition early enough so that a viable plan is available at discharge. This presents a particular problem for those children whose insurance permits only a very brief hospital stay (i.e., 3 to 4 weeks). Within these time limitations, it is difficult to evaluate the child and family, engage the parents in the decision-making process, and arrive at and implement a discharge plan. It is nevertheless essential that the process proceed as completely as possible.

The following dispositions are considered: return to the family with follow-up outpatient treatment plus special schooling where indicated, long-term residential treatment, foster care, and day treatment program.

Whenever possible, the child returns to his or her family. The staff works closely with the child and family during the hospitalization to assess how changes can be effected that would permit the child to remain in the home without the damaging interactions which led to the hospitalization. Lifelong family patterns cannot be restructured during a period of brief hospitalization; instead, one can only begin a therapeutic process. All children returning home need continued treatment for themselves and their families. The primary therapist helps the family arrange this either with him- or herself or with another therapist, either privately or through an appropriate psychiatric facility.

In addition to assessing the child's pathology, strengths, and responsiveness to treatment, the staff evaluates the family members' readiness and availability to involve themselves in an ongoing therapeutic process. The family's emotional resources and pathology are considered in disposition planning. The parents are helped to understand the child's problems and the importance of their role in helping the child progress. For example, the parent who fails to keep his or her own appointments with the therapist during the hospitalization or continually projects the blame for the child's difficulty onto the school or staff may not be very cooperative in outpatient treatment if the child were to go home. Conversely, a family which appears disorganized when the child is admitted into the hospital can demonstrate resources not evident in the beginning of the treatment.

L., for example, an immature 10-year-old boy, raised by his grandmother, presented serious problems in school. The grandmother infantilized and overstimulated him, and became very depressed when she had to separate from him for the hospitalization. Initially, the staff felt that the situation was intractable and that long-term residential placement would be needed. However, during the course of hospitalization, the grandparents regularly attended individual and family sessions with L.'s primary therapist and primary nurse and the grandmother regularly attended the parents' group. She mastered her problems with the separation and did not allow L. to manipulate her into taking him home prematurely. She began to recognize her needs to baby him and began to make some modifications in her interactions with him. Her ability to involve herself actively in the treatment process, and the shifts that were achieved in the interrelationships were indications that L. could make a successful adjustment at home with continued treatment for him and his family. One cannot emphasize enough the need to assess the parents and involve them as collaborators in the plan for the child and family. The child who does well in the hospital and has the ability to "make it" in the community may still need to go into residential treatment if the family cannot provide care and nurturing. At times, a homemaker can be used to provide support and structure for the family. Financial cutbacks in service often make this approach an unrealistic solution. If the parent does not want the child home and feels he or she cannot manage the child, the child's return home is bound to fail.

R., for example, a 12-year-old Puerto Rican boy, was hospitalized because of truanting, gang involvement, and mother's inability to control him. He was a bright, verbal, appealing youngster, who did extremely well on the inpatient unit. The staff felt that with outpatient treatment the child could return home. However, the mother remained fearful of the child's return home and throughout treatment favored placement. Her guilt over her wish to be rid of R. motivated her to agree to take him home. Shortly after discharge, the initial symptoms erupted and placement plans were initiated.

As much as the child and parents want the child to return home and have worked toward this end during the period of hospitalization, the actual discharge often produces anxiety and fear despite the insights and changes achieved. "The family and child both feel a sense of uncertainty as their reunion approaches" (Moss, 1968). The child is fearful that he or she will again be sent away and the parents worry that the symptoms would return when the child comes home. They feel inadequate and vulnerable in their parenting role. The therapist must be attended to these underlying feelings in order to help the parents and child master them prior to discharge.

Day and weekend passes are arranged in order that the child spend time in the home and neighborhood prior to discharge. Parents tend to arrange interesting outings during passes in order to compensate

for having placed the child in the hospital. The staff encourages the
family to simulate the real-life situation of the family. The family is
assigned tasks in order to test out new understandings and patterns
of relationships. The progress of the passes gives some indications
of the difficulties persisting which need to be dealt with in the posthospital treatment.

The planning for follow-up treatment needs to include posthospital
educational planning. Many of the children who require inpatient
treatment have had serious learning difficulties as well as behavior
problems at home or in school. Often a school is reluctant to readmit
a child because of the previous difficulties or because of a lack of
suitable class placement. Long bureaucratic delays are often encountered
in getting a special class placement within the public school system or
in a private school. Thus, the child may be without schooling for a
period of time following discharge. This is an added strain on both
parent and child. Twenty-four hour interaction between a disturbed
child and his troubled parents cannot be undone by once- or twice-a-
week treatment. Gains acheived in the hospital cannot be sustained
with such additional strain. It is essential to have a discharge plan
which avoids the child's being home without school.

Once the child is placed in school, the therapist and school need
to work closely together. The feedback from the school is a valuable
barometer for the therapist in the assessment of the child's progress.
Schools appreciate input from the therapist to help them deal with
the child more effectively. For example, during discussions with the
counselor of a special school it became clear that all of the children
referred for inpatient treatment from that school had auditory perceptual
problems. The school utilized this information not only in relation to
the children they had referred, but also in relation to their total
classroom population.

Although one of the goals of hospital treatment is to bring about a
beginning understanding and change in child and family so as to permit
the child to return home, this is not always possible. Many children
cannot return home immediately because of their or their family's
pathology and treatment needs. These children need the continued
intensity of a therapeutic milieu to support their fragile internal organization. They may be dangerous to themselves or others or have
extremely poor impulse control requiring continued protection of a
structured setting. They may have home situations that are too unstable
or parents too uninvolved to help them make a successful adjustment
at home.

During the period of hospitalization, the staff carefully observes
and evaluates parent/child interactions in order to assess the family's
availability and motivation for change. Parents who consciously or
unconsciously foster the child's pathology, are too beset by their own
reality or emotional problems, or are unavailable for involvement with
the staff on behalf of their child will have difficulty helping the child
to progress at home. Residential treatment may be indicated in these
situations. Such placement is a temporary situation with the aim of
continuing the work begun in the hospital so that the child can ultimately
return home.

For most parents, the recommendation for residential treatment
arouses considerable guilt and a feeling that they are "putting their
child away" or "giving him away." Even though the parent may recognize
the need and benefit of placement, he or she may be against placement
as a defense against ambivalent feelings toward the child. Most
children feel abandoned. They are acutely aware of any unconscious

wish by the parents to be rid of them. Most see themselves as having
been hospitalized because they are "bad" and placement is viewed
as a further punishment for their badness. Whenever long-term placement is considered, the plan is discussed with the family early enough
during the hospitalization to allow time for the parents and child to
work through their complex feelings. *"The family and child may react
to the coming separation with a great deal of anxiety...If they repress
these feelings, the trauma which comes with the actual separation may
be intensified"* (Moss, 1968).

The issue of placement is discussed in both individual and group
sessions. It is often the focus of both the community meeting and the
parents' group. Parents are able to offer each other considerable
support because they share ambivalent and guilt feelings. For example,
for two mothers the parents' group became a major vehicle for expressing
and sharing feelings and coming to terms with the decision for
residential treatment. One mother favored residential treatment, as she
recognized the continued treatment needs of her son; the other was
adamantly opposed. Discussion in parents' group and the work of
individual sessions helped both parents accept placement. Both boys
were to go to the same facility on the same date. The parents
supported each other throughout the separation, and were grateful for
each other's presence. One cannot underestimate how difficult a
decision this can be for parents and how much support they need from
the therapist and others during this time. Nor can one underestimate
the meaning of continued separation from parents for the child. A
great deal of therapeutic work must be done around this issue.

For some parents and children the decision for placement appears to
be an easier one. Some parents request residential treatment as soon
as the child is hospitalized because they are unable to deal with the
child or are frightened by his or her behavior or by the feelings they
experience which are aroused by the child's behavior. Similarly, many
children who feel out of control or recognize the lack of nurturing
provided by their environment welcome placement and the continued
care and structure. Some parents are frightened by the verbal and
physical abuse they have inflicted on their children. Even though the
parent-child relationship inevitably improves while the child is in the
hospital, the parent may remain fearful of their loss of control when
the child returns home. Continued placement is a safer option until
both child and parents solidify their gains.

R., a 5-year-old boy, was hospitalized because of extreme hyperactivity, his mother's inability to control him, and a potentially abusive
situation. His mother decided to bring the child for an inpatient
evaluation after an episode in which she hit him so hard as to leave
marks on his face. She was frightened by how angry and frustrated
he made her feel. During the course of hospitalization, visits and passes
went reasonably well, but she became frightened at the slightest
indication of his earlier problematic behavior. She requested residential
treatment not only because she felt her son needed further help but
also because she had not sufficiently mastered her own anger at his
behavior and was afraid that she would hurt him.

Another group of parents who more readily accept placement are
those who, for all intents and purposes, have already abandoned their
child. These parents rarely visit their children despite efforts to
involve them during the period of hospitalization. In some of these
situations, the Division of Children's Services has investigated possible
child abuse or severe neglect. Although these parents appear to
accept and even request placement the therapist must be aware of the

complexity of emotions aroused by placing a child and remain attuned to the underlying feelings of ambivalence and guilt. These feelings may in fact be heightened, albeit in a disguised form, when the parents themselves request the placement. Children who are essentially abandoned need to be placed as soon as practical in order to prevent an overattachment to the unit as their new home.

Children are referred to a wide range of residential treatment centers. The staff becomes acquainted with these facilities via field visits in order to select intelligently the one best suited to a child and family's needs. The family feels reassured when the therapist has some firsthand knowledge about the place to which the child is being referred.

It is sometimes difficult for the staff to recommend residential treatment, particularly when the child is very young and needs individual care. As an alternative, foster care rarely offers the child an ideal family who can provide care and nurturing while tolerating and understanding the deviant behavior. In these instances, the staff members must be aware of their own feelings and the conscious or unconscious message that is conveyed to the parents and child. The staff's ambivalence about placement may prevent them from helping the family members resolve their own ambivalent feelings about the placement of the child.

As with school plans, residential placement plans need to be made as early as possible in the child's hospitalization to allow time to work through the recommendation, and to work toward implementation as quickly from the hospital to ensure continuity of treatment. If this is not possible it is essential that outpatient treatment be offered during the interim period because of the continued stress to the family.

Some parents cannot accept a recommendation for residential placement because of their guilt. It may be necessary for them to reexperience the child at home and recognize their continued inability to manage the child. Mrs. D., the mother of a 12-year-old boy requested hospitalization for her son because of his behavioral difficulties and her inability to control him. At the outset, she requested placement. During the course of hospitalization, he improved, demonstrating none of his earlier deviant behavior. There had not been sufficient change in D. or in his poorly structured home environment to sustain the change; long-term residential treatment was recommended. Despite many discussions, D.'s mother saw the improvement as permanent and was unable to accept the recommendation. As the final decision was hers to make, she took him home. After a short stay at home, D.'s behavior deteriorated, and the mother was then able to agree on a placement plan for him.

Prior to a child's placement, the child and parents are interviewed at the residential treatment center. A staff member accompanies them to support them, answer questions for the facility, and deal with the parents' and child's ambivalences that may arise when actually confronted with the reality of continued separation. Most residential treatment centers agree with the philosophy that it is important to actively involve the parents in the final decision regarding admission to long-term placement.

It is clear that placing or treating the child is not a solution to the family's or child's problem. The treatment plan must include work with the family, since the vast majority of children eventually do return home. They may not be able to sustain treatment gains if changes have not occurred within the family as well. "The basic purpose of residential and day programs for troubled children should be to function as a family support system, rather than to treat the child in isolation from his family and home community" (Whittaker, 1975). This has been an area of concern when children do go into placement. Too often, inadequate resources preclude intensive work with families. This is recognized by residential treatment centers and more and more of them offer ongoing services to parents.

Foster care is another option available at the time the child is discharged from the hospital. It is usually difficult for biological parents to accept a recommendation for foster care because of the implication that another person is a better parent for their child. Residential treatment is often a more neutral, less threatening solution to parents. Residential treatment provides a transition for both child and parents if the child does eventually require foster care.

Many children who come to the hospital from foster care have been in a home where problems erupted. Foster agencies will often request an inpatient evaluation of a child in order to determine whether another foster home or another form of care is best for the child. Often, foster parents refuse to have the child back in their home because of the child's previous behavior. Even if the child cannot return to his foster parents, the staff attempts to involve the foster family in the treatment and planning for the child. At times the foster family may be the only family the child has ever known. Their continued involvement can help mitigate the child's feelings of being abandoned during hospitalization. Foster parents often know more about the child than the agency personnel and therefore can provide invaluable information. Similar to biological and adoptive parents, foster parents may feel that they have failed as parents. Understanding the child's illness and what may have gone wrong can be of great value to the family.

In order to decide whether a child can return to foster care, it is essential to evaluate the circumstances leading to the child's removal from the home. One needs to understand the degree to which the behavioral difficulties are reactive to the foster family or stimulated by the child's own internal pathology. In situations where the child's pathology creates great disturbances in the family, one can generally assume that similar situations would arise should the child return to another foster home. It is the rare foster home that can tolerate the degree of pathology that severely disturbed children may demonstrate. Foster parents need positive feedback from the child in order to sustain their involvement. If, on the other hand, the behavioral problems arise primarily out of interactions within the foster family, it is possible that with support and treatment the child would make an adequate adjustment in a carefully selected foster home. There is generally an interaction between the child's pathology with the foster family's behavior pattern and it may be very difficult to assess the contribution of each partner to the eruption of symptoms.

Those children who have already been in two or three foster homes before hospitalization pose a particularly difficult problem. They try to master their feelings of rejection by attempting to provoke rejection. This behavior is usually very difficult for a foster family to tolerate. Thus, a new foster home is likely to end as another failure and rejection for the child. It is often best that these children go into a residential treatment situation prior to going to another foster home. This allows them the opportunity to master their feelings of rejection by parental figures in a more neutral, less intense environment.

Similar to other dispositions, foster care must be planned well in advance so the child can go to his or her new home upon leaving the hospital. It is essential that the child meet the foster family and spend some time together with them prior to discharge. The foster family visits with the child in the hospital and is permitted to take the child to the new home on passes.

The formation of the day treatment program at Mount Sinai Medical Center was a result of the difficulties encountered in implementing adequate disposition plans for the children because of delays in placement and school planning. A day treatment program offers appropriate schooling and continued intensive treatment for the child and family. For the child awaiting placement, a day treatment program can provide continued support and treatment for the child and family during a period of heightened stress.

In summary, the essentials of posthospital planning involve careful and thorough assessment of the child and family, early planning with family involvement, helping the child and the family understand and accept the recommendations, making an adequate interim plan when required, and, as much as possible, implementing the disposition plan immediately following discharge to ensure continuity of treatment.

REFERENCES

Kemp, C.J. (1971). Family treatment within the milieu of a residential treatment center. *Child Welfare 50:* 229-235.
Mandelbaum, A. (1962). Parent-child separatum: Its significance to parents. *Soc. Work,* Oct., pp. 26-34.
Moss, S.Z. (1968). Integration of the family into the child placement process. *Children Today 15:* 219-224.
Whittaker, J.K. (1975). The ecology of child treatment: A developmental/ educational approach to the therapeutic milieu. *J. Aut. Childh. Schiz.* 5: 223-237.

Chapter 15

THE DAY TREATMENT PROGRAM

Christine Johns

Day treatment programs for emotionally disturbed children are a relatively recent development in the mental health field. The first North American day program developed within a traditional hospital was established in Montreal by Cameron in 1946. Historically, "psychiatric units in general hospitals were handicapped by three traditional medical characteristics: (a) a hospital is a place to go to bed, (b) a patient stays until he is well, and (c) only the patient is treated" (Glasscote et al., 1969, p. 1). Day programs allow the patient to be treated within the context of the family.

Prior to the existence of day treatment for emotionally disturbed children, children who required more intensive treatment than outpatient psychotherapy were referred to residential treatment centers. "While residential treatment is undoubtedly necessary for certain children, questions arise about the wisdom of removing young children from their families, for in the final analysis, children must adjust to a home and the social community" (LaVietes, Hulse, and Blau, 1960). The impetus for the development of the day treatment program at Mount Sinai Medical Center was a growing awareness that an intermediate facility between inpatient, outpatient, and residential treatment was lacking for the children discharged from the inpatient unit.

Many children who improve with hospital treatment return to a home situation which cannot provide enough structure and support to sustain the progress. Even with outpatient treatment and special schooling, symptomatology may recur. The day program was designed in order to provide a support system for these children and their families in several ways: (1) as an alternative to inpatient treatment or residential treatment, (2) as a transition between inpatient treatment and return to public school, (3) as preparation for residential treatment, (4) as supportive treatment through an after-school group, and (5) as short-term crisis intervention.

Since its inception in March, 1977, the day program has evolved into two components, the Day Treatment Program (DTP) and the After-School Program (ASP). The DTP services approximately eight children and their families and the ASP six. All the children are within the ages of 6 to 12 years. The eventual goal is to service 20 to 24 children and their families. The socioeconomic makeup is 85 percent Hispanic, Medicaid-funded patients. The remaining 15 percent are black and

Caucasian, and include Medicaid patients and a few who pay a sliding-scale fee. The average length of stay is 6 months to 1 year, with some children continuing in the ASP after discharge from the DTP.

The facility is presently housed in a large room located in an annex to the hospital. Other rooms within the hospital are available for lunch and gym. Renovations for a larger, better designed area have been delayed because of hospital administrative problems. In fact, many day programs face a variety of administrative problems including the use of whatever space is available for them rather than specifically designed units (Critchley and Berlin, 1979; Glassocte et al., 1969).

The DTP provides a full day of school and therapeutic activities. The children are involved in a special education class and a variety of sensori-motor, therapy, and activity groups. They participate in psychotherapy sessions, family meetings, parent-child activities, play group sessions, and community meetings each week. Lunch is provided by the hospital and bus transportation by the Board of Education. Medications are administered, if needed.

The ASP provides a supportive environment for children who are able to maintain themselves in public school but who have emotional, learning, and family problems. The activities are designed to improve impulse control, self-image, perceptual ability, and socialization skills. A parent-child activity is conducted once a week, in order to help parents and children improve their communication with each other. Parents and children may be seen individually, if indicated. The ASP meets each afternoon for 1 hour and the family arranges transportation. During the summer, the DTP and ASP are combined to form one group which is primarily activity oriented.

Administratively, the day program functions under the supervision of the inpatient unit. The primary staff consists of two registered nurses, one of whom (a senior clinical nurse) is the coordinator of the program, an occupational therapist, and a special education teacher. Second-year child psychiatry fellows serve as consultants and participate in part of the group and activity therapy program. Volunteers, students, and staff members from the inpatient unit are utilized to provide a variety of role models for the children. Staff training and supervision is provided via the administrative structure of the inpatient unit.

Patient treatment plans are periodically reassessed and formally discussed every 2 weeks in conferences which are attended by the child psychiatry fellows, the attending child psychiatrist, social workers, the clinical nursing supervisor, and the primary DTP staff. Daily notes are written according to the problem-oriented model and reviewed during the conferences. The responsibilities of the treatment team includes: (1) the completion of a full evaluation for each child and family; (2) the formulation and implementation of individualized treatment plans; (3) providing ongoing critical evaluation of the therapeutic value of the program; (4) the establishment of effective lines of communication with other members of the team, with community agencies, and with the public school system; and (5) the creation of a caring atmosphere where growth is stimulated and health is fortified.

Children who have learning difficulties with associated problems such as hyperactivity, symbiotic relationships, language and thought disorders, poor impulse control, organicity, character disorders, autistic features, depression, school phobias, and unsocialized aggressive reactions have been found to respond effectively in the DTP or ASP. Severely retarded, severely autistic, and uncontrollably aggressive children require a more protective environment then the day program can offer and may need to be away from home.

The program's philosophical approach stresses the developmental progression of the child and family. "Child treatment programs should focus on growth and development in the child's total life sphere, rather than on the amelioration of psychiatrically defined syndromes or the extinction of certain problematic behaviors" (Whittaker, 1975). Whittaker emphasizes teaching children skills for living while they participate in a day program. The therapeutic milieu provides a "multidimensional context for competency acquisition where the events of daily living—the rules, the routines, the games and activities, the psychotherapy, and the classroom education – become not just the context for helping a child manage his behavior, but a medium for helping him to expand his competence to the full limits of his developmental potential" (p. 231).

In order to understand the child and help his or her developmental progression, the staff needs to work with the other family members. Many of the families are chaotic, unstable, and experience repeated life crises. Thus, the day program has become a family-centered treatment facility whose primary objective is accomplished by teaching families methods of coping with their child's problems. The needs of other family members are recognized and home visits occur when appropriate. The parents are seen individually and conjointly with the child in verbal and/or activity sessions.

A major focus is the child's education. Learning difficulties and perceptual problems are evaluated and the child is helped to compensate for his or her deficits so that frustration does not overwhelm the willingness to learn. Classwork is assigned according to the level of each child's ability and progression to the next higher level is supported and rewarded. The children's education includes learning academic skills in the classroom as well as learning how to function in the everyday world. The DTP and ASP thus provide a socialization experience for the children. The vehicles include therapeutic groups such as community meetings, play groups, activities-of-daily-living group, and activity skills groups. The children learn how to communicate more effectively with each other as well as with adults. Ego interpretations by the staff, peer pressure, and the use of rewards allow the children to enhance their social skills.

The use of behavior modification techniques evolved as the result of a need for structure and limits while providing for positive reinforcement for socially appropriate behavior and skill attainment. Because of the physical limitations and the nature of the day program, it is difficult to enforce limits in the same way that they can be enforced on an inpatient unit. Children cannot be easily removed from the classroom when they become disruptive. Time-outs are encouraged by the staff before the child loses control. The fundamentals of behavior modification provide an incentive to complete classwork, to participate in activities, to talk out disturbing feelings rather than act out, and to gain a sense of achievement through goal attainment. Both group and individual "programs" have been designed whereby the children receive daily rewards according to a graduated scale of points which can be traded for objects from a "store" at the end of each day.

A variety of circumstances led to a program design whereby the primary staff of the DTP, that is, the nurses and occupational therapist, function as primary therapists for most of the children and families. The psychotherapy and family work is thus an extension of the work accomplished in the rest of the milieu. Lack of formal training in individual and family psychotherapy has been compensated by on-site, ongoing supervision by the attending child psychiatrist.

Issues of transference and countertransference are dealt with frequently. In fact, after experiencing these phenomena in individual sessions, the staff has become more cognizant of their importance in the treatment of the children in the general milieu.

The treatment of a particular mother and her two children included weekly family sessions. This mother was extremely infantile and clearly favored the younger sibling because the older one reminded her of her ex-husband. The father would visit periodically and take the boys on trips. In the supervisory discussions it became clear that the mother felt criticized by the therapist's statements and actions. This was a transference feeling connected to her feeling that when the father visited the boys, he acted as if he was a better parent. In the same way, she feared that the therapist would act like a better parent. Clarification of these issues led to an elaboration of the family dynamics. The mother infantilized the younger child and teased the older child, who in turn teased the younger one who then misbehaved. The mother was able to understand these connections and discuss how she treated the older son as if he was the hated father.

In conclusion, day treatment for emotionally disturbed children is a valuable therapeutic modality which can be provided as the primary form of treatment or as an intermediate stage during a child's course of treatment. Family involvement "permits simultaneous growth of child and parents so that readjustment is a continuous and not a sudden process" (LaVietes et al., 1964, p. 168). Since not all children with emotional illnesses are able to respond to day treatment, a careful screening procedure is needed. Day treatment consists of a tripartite program: (1) psychotherapeutic interventions with the child, (2) psychotherapeutic interventions with the family, and (3) remedial education.

REFERENCES

Critchley, D.L., and Berlin, I.N. (1979). Day treatment of young psychotic children and their parents. *Child. Psychia. Hum. Dev.* 9: 227-237.

Glasscote, R.M., Kraft, A.M., Glassman, S.M., and Jepson, W.W. (1969). *Partial Hospitalization for the Mentally Ill.* Washington, D.C.: American Psychiatric Association.

LaVietes, R., Cohen, R., Reens, R., and Ronall, R. (1965). Day treatment center and school: Seven years experience. *Am. J. Orthopsychiatry* 35: 160-169.

LaVeites, R., Hulse, W.C., and Blau, A. (1960). A psychiatric day treatment center and school for young children and their parents. *Am. J. Orthopsychiatry* 30: 468-482.

Whittaker, J.K (1975). The ecology of child treatment: A developmental/ educational approach to the therapeutic milieu. *J. Aut. Childh. Schiz.* 5: 223-237.

Chapter 16

THE COMMUNITY MEETING—A PARADIGM
OF MILIEU THERAPY

Leon Hoffman
Mary Ann Wagner

The backbone of most therapeutic milieus or therapeutic communities is the patient-staff or community meeting. The process and content of this meeting reflects the atmosphere and organization of the milieu and the culture of the community is transmitted to newly arrived members. The literature deals extensively with the utilization of a community meeting in the treatment of adult psychiatric patients (Almond, 1974) as well as with group psychotherapy for children (Slavson and Schiffer, 1975), yet there is limited material regarding the role, function, and value of a community meeting in the psychiatric treatment of children in inpatient, day, or residential centers.

Bender (1937) describes how group discussions help the hospitalized child deal with a variety of issues. Redl (1959a) introduced the concept of the life space interview, whereby asocial behavior is confronted directly while underlying feelings are elicited, accepted, and understood.

Nearly every program that concerns itself with the treatment of emotionally disturbed children schedules a variety of meetings in which the staff and children participate. Such meetings serve crucial unifying and stabilizing functions in the organization of the program.

The community meeting is a paradigm for such meetings. A community which includes severely disturbed children can be closely knit and tension-filled. There is a conglomeration of individuals, staff and children, who are interdependent and influence one another. The community meeting is vital because it provides a forum where critical unit issues can be brought into the open, discussed, and problem solving begun.

The social structure, emotional climate, and group dynamics of the unit are observable in a community meeting. The relationships and interactions among the staff, between staff and children, and among the children themselves can be observed. Other phenomena that can be observed include scapegoating and clique formation (Redl, 1959b), order or chaos, organization or disorganization, tension, depression, or anxiety. Potential problems may be discussed at a meeting before they are manifested in other areas. They can be confronted and escalation of anxiety prevented.

A community meeting is quite different from group psychotherapy, yet a knowledge of group dynamics and techniques is mandatory for the effective management of the meeting. Many more people are involved than in group psychotherapy; a community meeting is much more structured. Group psychotherapy is more apt to eventually deal with deeper dynamic issues; the interplay between the staff and children is much more complex in a community meeting because so many staff and children are in attendance. The leader of the meeting needs to be attuned to the many possible factors that may be operative. At the same time, the other staff need to feed back to the leader issues that he or she may overlook.

As has been described previously (Chap. 2), the milieu and group aspects of the Mount Sinai Medical Center Child Psychiatry Inpatient Unit have been strengthened enormously over the past years. This chapter describes the genesis and development of the community meeting which coincides with the development of the milieu and group program.

Prior to 1974, the major psychotherapeutic group work on the unit consisted of a three times a week, 20- to 30-minute morning meeting. The child psychiatry fellows, the day nursing staff, and all the children attended these meetings. The group leadership was rotated among the child fellows (several months at a time). Occasionally, when there were several young children on the unit, a play group was formed as a substitute for the regular meeting, a talking group. The main purpose of these groups was to obtain information to facilitate the psychiatric fellows and social workers in the individual psychotherapy with the children and casework with their families. The benefit in terms of unit management and milieu treatment was of secondary importance. This arrangement continued until 1975. At that time the focus of the unit changed. The nursing staff began to take a more active positive role via the implementation of primary nursing. The milieu, group, and school programs were seen to be as crucial as the individual and family treatment to the overall treatment of the child and family.

It became apparent that the group psychotherapy program needed reorganization. The children were divided into two groups rather than one large morning group. One was a talking group for the older children and the other a play group for the younger, early latency-age group (see Chap. 9 and Abramson, Hoffman, and Johns, 1979). The length of these meetings was increased to 45 minutes and the frequency decreased to twice a week. The two groups functioned more effectively and were more therapeutic. However, the lack of an integrated approach soon became apparent. The staff became cognizant of the need for a formal meeting attended by most of the staff and all of the children to help improve the management of the children's day-to-day living experience.

A series of events during the winter holiday season of 1975 clearly dramatized the lack of an integrated milieu program. The Department of Nursing was in the process of administrative reorganization, creating tension and insecurity. There was only one child psychiatry fellow assigned to the unit at the time, placing an inordinate burden of responsibility on everyone. These factors led to disorder and demoralization among the staff and children. The patient population included several aggressive preadolescents. As an example of the staff disorganization, episodes of physical aggression directed toward the staff by one 12-year-old girl were not confronted directly. Another preadolescent girl was precipitously discharged to a residential treatment center 2 days before Christmas because the responsible social agency was unable to obtain a court order to extend her hospital stay. The unit staff took a passive stance. The Christmas season itself was a

further catalyst leading to a sequence of dangerous acts by the patients,
such as breaking windows. Two of the children were administratively
discharged for the safety of the others on the unit. These events
illustrate how staff disorganization leads to disorganization among the
children. The staff feels helpless and some children may then become
scapegoats.

A series of urgent meetings were conducted in an effort to confront
the crisis, to begin to unify the staff, and to convey to the children
a sense of cohesiveness which would increase their feelings of
security. These meetings were held during the lunch hour with staff
members positioning themselves among the children and discussing the
problem behaviors. As a result of this upheaval, numerous candid
discussions among the staff led to a reorganization that created an
effective therapeutic team approach. The community meeting evolved
from these lunchtime crisis meetings. Resolution of the crisis resulted
in an effective team structure and a stronger milieu and group program.

Initially the community meeting was held in the morning. In order
to include the evening nursing staff in some of the daytime activities,
the meeting time was changed to the late afternoon. The community
meeting is now consistently held every Wednesday throughout the year
for a period of 30 minutes. In attendance are all the children, day
nursing staff on duty, one or two of the evening nursing staff, the
occupational and activity therapist, the child psychiatry fellows, the
supervisory social worker, and the psychiatrist in charge of the unit.
A member of the nursing staff, usually the day senior clinical nurse,
is the leader of the meeting.

The community meeting is conducted in the lounge with the chairs
arranged in one large circle. A variety of arrangements have been
attempted, including the use of tables and serving snacks. One large
circle is most effective. In this manner, the leader is able to maintain
control of the meeting and all the members of the group are visible to
one another. Prior to the meeting the children and some of the staff
arrange the chairs. The leader meets briefly with other staff prior
to the meeting in order to review the specific issues that may be affecting
the community, that is, the announcements that are to be made, the unit
tone, and any other significant themes that may have an effect on the
children and staff. It is crucial for the staff, especially the leader, to
be aware of pertinent events, as demonstrated by the following
experience.

The children were anxious, agitated, and resistant to allow the
meeting to begin; one preadolescent girl refused to join the meeting.
A staff member finally remembered that this patient had exposed herself
in school that afternoon. When this behavior was verbalized for the
children, they were able to talk about the anxiety generated by the
girl's behavior.

A major function of the community meeting is the announcement of
events that affect the entire unit: admissions, discharges, staff vacations,
school holidays, upcoming events, and behaviors affecting the community,
that is, aggression, sex play, scapegoating. The meeting begins with
the leader making all the announcements. Then, one of the children is
asked to explain the purpose of the meeting and its rules to the new-
comers. The remainder of the session is often structured around the
issue announced. If all the announcements are not made at the beginning,
the session is often complicated by a tangential discussion that may not
be crucial for the homeostasis of the unit. Whenever there is resistance
among the staff and/or children to openly discuss an anxiety-provoking
issue such as a staff member's leaving or the bizarre behavior of a

psychotic or retarded child, an important announcement may be omitted completely or mentioned at the end of the meeting. Premeeting preparation coupled with delaying in-depth discussion until after all announcements have been made ensures that the most important issues will be stated early and adequately ventilated.

A community activity conducted by one therapeutic activities and one nursing staff member follows the community meeting. The activity is a transition period which allows the children a nonverbal, symbolic medium to deal with the issues raised in the meeting. At the conclusion of the community meeting the occupational therapist describes the proposed activity. The activity chosen usually reflects the theme of the meeting. For example, if the theme has been separation, the children often play a game such as "scavenger hunt" or "hot-and-cold" in order to help promote their mastery of this issue; for the theme of sibling rivalry, a community mural or a group sing-along promotes the reaction-formation of togetherness and cooperation. A particularly innovative activity involves making name stickers for the rooms when the children are concerned about lack of privacy and sexual overstimulation.

Since the number of people who attend the community meeting is quite large (12 to 14 children and about 16 adults) and the topics discussed are frequently anxiety-producing, a careful structure has proved to be mandatory in order to conduct a therapeutic meeting, that is, one that decreases anxiety, increases cohesiveness among the children and staff, and allows for verbalization of feelings without aggression. With increasing experience, it has become clear that a "structured-spontaneous" meeting format is most effective.

As part of the structure the children are obliged to sit within the circle and are not allowed to fight with or provoke one another. They identify with the staff and, in a sense, learn that talking about feelings is helpful whereas fighting or provoking is harmful. During one week, for example, three boys had been physically aggressive towards a female psychiatry fellow. During the meeting there was an obvious under-current of anxiety; the fellow's name was mentioned in whispered, angered tones, loud enough to be heard. At this point the leader made a statement about the incident. The staff communicated to the children that everyone has feelings of anger and rage at various times in life. The effective way to deal with these feelings is by talking in whatever words one chooses to use, but fighting cannot be permitted or tolerated. Initially there was silence, then laughing and silliness, until the children realized that indeed they could talk about what had happened without fear of punishment.

If a child cannot abide by the minimal rules, the leader asks the child to take a time-out (in the hallway) and to return to the meeting when he or she is able to conform to the expected behavior. When a child is unable to take time-out (mainly because of aggression), the leader will ask another staff member to accompany the child out of the meeting. At the end of the meeting the leader announces and praises the children who were able to participate in the meeting.

It has become quite clear that when the staff becomes less ambivalent about the importance of rules in order to maintain the necessary limits, it is rare that any child will need more than an occasional time-out.

The problem of separation is often a central theme. Bender (1937) stressed the importance of group discussions to help hospitalized children deal with the uncertainties of their disposition. The children are affected in various ways by the theme of separation: recently admitted children are often homesick and not an integral part of the community, children about to be discharged face the loss of important attachments on the unit, some face the unpredictability of a new environment, and some children are unsure of what will happen after hospitalization. Very importantly, the children regard the vacations taken by their nurse, therapist, and other staff members as significant losses and abandonments.

The community meeting has proved to be a valuable tool for the education of all staff. An important principle in the milieu treatment of emotionally disturbed children is the interrelationship among the various activities, groups, meetings, and sessions. The community meeting is a microcosm of the unit. The themes that are discussed during this meeting are usually elaborated in the individual sessions, other groups, activities, and general milieu.

In contrast to other groups and activities conducted on the unit, many adults participate in the community meeting. In the other groups and activities, the two or three staff members who participate can work together with a high degree of mutual collaboration. This kind of collaboration is very difficult at a meeting where there are often more adults than children. Staff members may differ as to what is the most crucial issue or what is or is not inappropriate behavior requiring limit-setting. Some staff feel insecure and fear exposing themselves at the meeting by "saying or doing the wrong thing." As a result of this, many staff do not participate actively but remain quiet.

The staff has to learn both the general function of the meeting as well as the role and function of the individual staff member. The staff needs to bring to the leader's and group's attention any perception (about) the issues discussed. They need to voice their opinions about a disruptive child requiring a time-out. The leader of the meeting decides which issue to discuss and whether or not a time-out is needed. In this way all staff members are encouraged to participate. Whenever more staff do actively participate the meeting is more therapeutic.

Staff dissatisfaction is often a result of a lack of understanding of the value of an activity. Increased staff participation and decreased dissatisfaction is achieved by educating the various staff members as to their role and function. This is accomplished via a brief wrap-up discussion after the community meeting, weekly discussions about the various groups on the unit, and individual discussions.

A community meeting, like a unit in general, involves an ongoing dynamic process dependent upon the vicissitudes of staff interrelationships as well as the changing population of children. As an educational tool, the meeting provides a forum whereby staff at all levels can view the children's behavior, begin to understand its meaning, and apply this understanding in the treatment of the general milieu. The community meeting provides and maintains a framework for the therapeutic environment for the treatment of the children. It can provide an impetus for increasing insight into the staff members' reactions to each other and to the children by receiving feedback from others. The meeting and the discussions about the meeting provide a structure and organization within which the various levels of staff are able to develop. In general terms the community meeting is a therapeutic process that aids in decreasing anxiety and helps to increase cohesiveness among the staff as well as the children.

REFERENCES

Abramson, R., Hoffman, L., and Johns, C. (1979). Play group for
    early latency age children on a short-term psychiatric unit. *Int.*

*J. Group Psychother. 29:*383-392.

Almond, R. (1974). *The Healing Community.* New York:Aronson.

Bender, L. (1937). Group activities on a children's ward as methods of psychotherapy. *Am. J. Psychiatry 93:*1151-1173.

Redl, F. (1959a). Life space interview techniques. *Am. J. Orthopsychiatry 29:*1-18.

Redl, F. (1959b). The concept of a therapeutic milieu. *Am. J. Orthopsychiatry 29:*721-736.

Slavson, S.R., and Schiffer, M. (1975). *Group Psychotherapies for Children.* New York: Int. Univ. Press.

AFTERWORD

Leon Hoffman

Many of the children treated at the Mount Sinai Medical Center
Inpatient and day treatment programs can be described, as did Kernberg,
as having borderline conditions.* These children have severe symptoms
and difficulties, disturbances in the development of their sense of self,
disturbances in the development of object relations, difficulties in
modulating their affects, and deficits in their ego functions.

The problem of long-term treatment for these children is crucial.
Since they have a difficult time learning from experience, a simple
supportive educational approach would seem to be inadequate. The
Psychotherapy Research Project of the Menninger Foundation indicated
that borderline patients responded best to supportive, expressive
modes of treatment rather than to simply supportive therapies.

The aim of the treatment program on the inpatient unit and the
day treatment program is to begin to help the children establish stable
self-concepts, increase their reality testing, and facilitate adequate
sublimations to help the progress of their development. This goal is
accomplished not simply by a psychoanalytically oriented psychotherapy,
nor by a supportive/educational approach, but by the multimodal team
approach described in this volume.

One can judge the validity of Kernberg's statement that these
children do not learn from experience via the clinical observation that
those who seem to do best are the ones who can become involved in
very long-term, intense therapeutic treatment programs. A significant
number of children who do go to residential treatment centers do well
while in residence but experienced renewed difficulties when they
return home.

This is an important mental health and social problem. These
children form the population from which delinquents and other troubled
adolescents and adults arise. Many of the residential treatment centers
to which the children go after hospitalization or after a time in the day
program provide mainly supportive and educational services plus a
varying amount of individual, group, and family psychotherapy. Many
children do respond to this approach.

However, for many others, a supportive approach is but a respite
on the road to more florid psychopathology. The approach described
in this book is obviously expensive. One needs to evaluate the efficacy

of the use of long-term treatment in a milieu where there is an integration of developmental and psychodynamic issues. Many trained staff, plus time for staff development and communication, are required to make such a program effective. This approach would foster internalization of new values by the child to allow for developmental progression.

From a monetary point of view, one can see that an investment early in a child's life, *if* it is effective, undoubtedly saves money in the long run. From the individual's and society's point of view, clinical research is still required as to what is the best *long-term* approach for these severely disturbed children.

---

*Kernberg, P. (1977). Borderline conditions: Childhood and adolescent aspects. Presented to the Second Annual Combined Meeting of the Society for Adolescent Psychiatry with the New York Council on Child Psychiatry.

APPENDIX 1

INPATIENT SCREENING – MOUNT SINAI HOSPITAL
CHILD PSYCHIATRY

GENERAL:

Name_____Age____DOB_____Sex___

Address_____Relative's telephone_____ (family)

Ethnic group_____Religion_____

Unit #_____School_____Grade____Special class_____Yes___ No___

Date_____Evaluator_____

Referred by_____Phone_____Admission date_____

Insurance_____

FAMILY INFORMATION (Biological, unless noted)

Mother:

Name_____Age_____Education_____

Occupation_____Medical and psychiatric_____

Welfare   Yes____   No____

Illness and/or treatment_____

Trouble with law, alcoholism, drugs_____

Father:

Name_____Age_____Education_____

Occupation_____Medical and psychiatric_____

Welfare   Yes____   No___

Illness and/or treatment_____

Trouble with law, alcoholism, drugs_____

Siblings (Names, ages, education):

_____
_____
_____

Child's place in sibship:_____

Family's Socioeconomic Status (SES) (circle one):

   I, II, III, IV, V

Who lives at home: (Name all relatives and others. Note if any have medical or psychiatric illnesses.)

_____
_____
_____

CHIEF COMPLAINT (Duration, precipitating factors)

_____
_____

CURRENT SYMPTOMS (Rate According to: 0 = not present; 1 = mild;
2 = moderate; 3 = severe)

Use the following to indicate chronicity:
* acute symptom;
** chronic symptom;
*** past symptom not in present

Suicidal thoughts___
Suicidal acts___
Anxiety, fears, phobias,
obsessions, compulsions___
Depressed mood, inferiority___
Enuresis___
Sleep problem___
Somatic concerns, hypochondriasis___
Social withdrawal, isolation___
Dependency, clinging___
Grandiosity___
Suspicion, persecution___
Delusions___
Hallucinations___
Anger, belligerence negativism___
Homicidal gestures___
Assaultive acts___
Fighting at home___
Fighting at school___
Firesetting___
Cruelty to animals___

Stealing___
Elopement, running away___
Truancy___
Temper tantrums___
Trouble with law___
School suspension___
Alcohol abuse___
Sexual problems___
Narcotics, other drugs___
Antisocial attitudes___
Trouble relating with others___
Problem playing by himself___
Agitation, hyperactivity at home___
Agitation, hyperactivity at school___
Disorientation, impaired memory___
Trouble learning___
Speech disorganization, incoherence___
Slowed up, lack of emotion___
Inappropriate affect, appearance,
or behavior___
Daily routine, leisure time
impairment___

How is family coping with the problem?

_____
_____

DEVELOPMENT:
Pregnancy problems_____
Birthweight_____
Abnormal milestones or development_____
Seizures_____

PLAY:
What kinds of toys, or games, special activities, transitional objects
are used or engaged in?_____

Social Play (circle appropriate description):
Solitary, Parallel, Cooperative, Chum relationship

Quality (circle appropriate description):
Passive, Aggressive, Retarded, Other

Has TREATMENT been attempted? (Modality—where and when?):

_____
_____

Medical Problems:

_____
_____

Opinion about parents' interest:

_____
_____
_____

MENTAL STATUS

Appearance (check applicable description):
  Well Nourished___   Poorly Nourished___
  Well Developed___   Poorly Developed___
  Distractable   Yes___   No___
  Bizarre Behavior   Yes___   No___
  Dress: Neat___ Sloppy___ Unremarkable___

Activity: Restless___ Sedentary___ Hypoactive___

Attitude:
  Cooperative   Yes___   No___
  Friendly   Yes___   No___

Orientation:
  Time   Yes___   No___
  Place   Yes___   No___
  Person   Yes___   No___

Affects (Rate according to: 0 = none; 1 = mild; 2 = moderate; 3 = severe):
  Anxious   ___   Withdrawn___   Angry   ___
  Fearful   ___   Cheerful ___   Negativistic ___
  Suspicious___   Excited ___   Flat   ___
  Depressed___   Elated   ___

Appropriateness of Affect (Rate according to: 1 = appropriate; 2 = inappropriat
  To thought   ___
  To surroundings ___

  Labile affect: Yes___   No___

Speech (Check applicable description):
  Pressure: Increased___   Decreased___   Normal___
  Amount: Silent___   Unremarkable___   Overtalkative___
  Expression: Clear___   Slurred___   Not understood___
               Immature___

Stream of Thought – Association (Check applicable description):
  Unremarkable___   Loose___   Tangential___   Circumstantial___
  Distractable___

Thought Content:
  Delusions   Yes___   No___
  Hallucination   Yes___   No___
    (Specify_____)
  Obsessive   Yes___   No___
  Illogical   Yes___   No___
  Bizarre   Yes___   No___
  Incoherent   Yes___   No___
  Suicidal   Yes___   No___
  Homicidal   Yes___   No___
  Separation anxiety   Yes___   No___

  Memory: Intact_____   Impaired___

  Reading_____
  Arithmetic _____
  Goodenough_____
  Orientation of time sequence_____

CASE DETERMINATION

Disposition:_____Admit:_____MSH OPD Rx_____

Other:_____

Reason for Hospitalization:_____

Problems according to child psychiatry problem list:

Diagnosis:_____

TREATMENT PLAN (Be specific)

1. Primary staff
2. Groups
3. Milieu
4. Family
5. Education and cognitive
6. Physical
7. Sensori-motor

APPENDIX 2

PROBLEM-ORIENTED MEDICAL RECORD
PROBLEM LIST FORMAT FOR (POMR) FORMAT*

1. General Appearance:

    Mannerisms and habits – tics, gestures, twirling, posturing,
    nail biting, cough, rocking, banging, masturbating, rubbing,
    going to bathroom, hair pulling; physical deformities; abnormality
    in habitus; inappropriate clothing, repetitive acts; compulsive
    acts; large for age; small for age; attention span; distractability,
    frustration tolerance, other significant features.

2. Somatic Complaints and Symptoms:

    Enuresis, encopresis, asthma, bronchitis, stomach aches,
    headaches, vomitting, diarrhea, rhinorrhea, allergic symptoms,
    obesity, weight loss, anorexia, sleep problem, other physical
    ailments.

3. Motility and Coordination:

    a. Hyperkinetic, hypokinetic: Is there specific stimulus?
        Does it change and vary during different situations?
    b. Gross motor: Balance, gait, posture, hopping, associated
        movements, clumsiness.
    c. Fine motor: Tapping, smoothness in play, smoothness in
        writing, drawing, geometric forms (circle, square, triangle,
        diamond).
    d. Eye-hand dominance (telescope and pinpoint screen).

4. Speech and Language:

    Articulation, rhythm, rate, organization, syntax, (situation in
    which abnormality is perceived); mutism (elective, essential);
    stuttering; hearing (whisper, tuning fork, watch); sentence
    length; naming, finding, and knowledge of function of common
    objects – key, pencil, paper, watch, calendar, ring, etc.;
    following directions, commands, and conversations, etc.

5. Intellectual Functioning:

    Vocabulary, reading level and comprehension (oral gray
    paragraphs); arithmetic; judgment; quality of communication;
    spontaneity; poise, ability to complete tasks; knowledge of colors.

    Tests that can be used: Goodenough Scale (approximate mental
    age), House-Tree-Person; Bender-Gestalt; Drawing of family.

6. Thinking and Perception:

    Incoherence, irrelevancy, tangentiality, neologisms, echolalia,
    bizarre preoccupations, wandering thoughts, rushing thoughts,
    slowed thoughts, obsessions, phobic thoughts; hallucinations
    (auditory, visual, olfactory, tactile, gustatory) – (differentiate
    from obsessive thought); delusions; defense mechanisms. Ability
    to distinguish fantasy from reality – does fantasy deal with
    real-life wishes? Bizarre? Sexual? Is it replete with sadism?
    Megalomanic fantasies? Three wishes.

---

*Source: Goodman, J.D., and Sours, J.A. (1967). *The Child Mental
Status Examination.* New York: Basic Books.

6a.   Dreams and Nightmares:

Animals, witches, monsters, soliders, etc. Related to TV,
movies, other real experience. Symbolic dream or undisguised
concrete representation? Concept of time, space, body (include
drawing); suicidal or homicidal thoughts; concept of death –
permanent separation, reunion, continuation of life someplace
else, etc.

7.   Emotional Reactions:

Fear, anxiety, anger, sadness, shame, elation, hypomania,
grandiosity, lability, flatness. Secondary responses: apathy,
petulance, arbitrariness, sulking, docility, negativism, aggression,
belligerence, obstinacy; inappropriateness of response.

8.   Manner of relating:

(a) Separation from mother (or mothering person) and other
family: acts as if she no longer exists; separates easily with
some apprehension; separates with a lot of apprehension; refuses
to separate or has severe tantrums. (b) Relation to staff –
indifferent, passive, dependent, aggressive, hostile, suspicious,
manipulative, antiauthority, dramatic, friendly, trusting, with
physical contact, without eye contact, somnolent, withdrawal,
acts as if staff not present; hints of merging with staff. (c)
Relation to other children: inappropriate peer relations; lack of
cooperation; quality of interactions, etc.

9.   Character of Play:

Initiates spontaneously or responds to initial invitations; degree
of integration and organization; ability to complete task; sex
appropriateness; level of maturity; intensity of aggression,
content, etc.

10.   Family:

Reliability; understanding of child's and family's problems; overt
psychopathology; interactions among family members and with
designated patient; interactions with staff; manner of dealing
with child's hospitalization or placement (e.g., denial, projection
of guilt with belligerence, etc.).

APPENDIX 3

MOUNT SINAI MEDICAL CENTER –
CHILD PSYCHIATRY ROUTINE WORK-UP OUTLINE

1. Identifying Data: Name, age ethnic group, religion, sex, living situation, school, grade.

2. State of Problem: Referral.   Onset, complaints, and by whom.

3. History of Problem: Development in detail.

4. Past History:

   a. Birth and development: Course of pregnancy; delivery; birth weight; nursing (breast or bottle); sitting up; walking; talking; weaning; teething; sphincter training (anal, diurnal, enuresis, nocturnal enuresis).

   b. Past illnesses:
      (1) Infantile: Age and course of each.
      (2) Surgical: T & A, appendectomy, etc.
      (3) Traumatic: Fractures, accidents, etc.
      (4) Allergic: Skin; hayfever, foods, asthma, etc.

   c. Physiological: General health and development; height and weight; headaches; ears; nose; eyes; sinus illness; dental; sore throats and colds; appetite; food fads, abdominal complaints; constipation or diarrhea; nocturnal and diurnal frequency; skin condition (acne, eczema); muscle and joint conditions; menses (age of onset, period, dysmenorrhea, mood changes).

   d. Education: Nursery school; elementary; high school; difficult subjects, easy subjects; study habits; disabilities (reading, spelling, arithmetic); tardiness; school behavior; social relations with schoolmates; extracurricular activities.

   e. Personality:
      1.   Ambition and future plans (fill in):

      2.   Play: Type of play; quality; history of transitional object.

      3.   Interests and hobbies: Radio, TV; comics; reading; movies; special (stamps, models, dolls, cooking, etc.); athletics (ball, tennis, swimming, teams, etc.).

      4.   Social: Siblings; playmates (younger, same age, older); relatives; leader or follower; aggressive or passive; amiable or pugnacious; fighting capacity; competitiveness.

      5.   Sex: Masturbation (technique, fantasies, frequency, guilt); heterosexual or homosexual; sex information (from parents, others).

      6.   Character: Frustration tolerance; temper; cooperation; obedience; rebelliousness; jealously; envy; fears; tantrums; compulsions; obsessive trends; nail biting; stuttering; enuresis, amiability; crying; depressive trends.

5. Family:

   a. Siblings: (list in order of age); name; age; school; social and special relations to patient and parent.

   b. Father: Name; age; health; education; work history; marital history; personality, etc.

    c. Mother: Name; age; health; education; work history; marital history; personality, etc.

Indicate biological parents, foster parents, step parents, commonlaw, etc.

6. Mental Status: Appearance, behavior, somatic complaints and symptoms; mobility, coordination (fine and gross motor); speech, language, intellectual functioning (including Goodenough Draw-a-Person), thinking; perception, emotional reactions (moods and affects); manner of relating; quality and character of play.

7. General Physical Exams (fill in):

8. Special Neurological Exam (fill in):

9. Diagnostic Impression (This is tentative and may be changed in subsequent progress and discharge notes):

    a. Descriptive (fill in):
      (1) Behavior
      (2) Communication ability
      (3) Physical and medical
      (4) Developmental
      (5) Psychological
      (6) Cognitive
      (7) Family

    b. Psychodynamic Formulation and Character Structure (fill in):

    c. Problems (fill in):

    d. Treatment Plan:

APPENDIX 4

MOUNT SINAI MEDICAL CENTER –
CHILD PSYCHIATRY TREATMENT PLAN (INITIAL/REVISED)

NAME_____   DATE_____

STAFF PRESENT_____

Problems	Severity: 0=None; 1=Mild; 2=Moderate; 3=Severe	Significant change of status; treatment plan (include role of various disciplines)
1. Appearance	0 1 2 3	
2. Somatic	0 1 2 3	
3. Motility and Coordination	0 1 2 3	
4. Speech and Language	0 1 2 3	
5. Intellectual	0 1 2 3	
6. Thinking and Perception	0 1 2 3	
7. Emotional Reaction	0 1 2 3	
8. Relationships	0 1 2 3	
9. Play–Spontaneous, Structured	0 1 2 3	
10. Family	0 1 2 3	
11. Special Symptoms	0 1 2 3	
12. Disposition	0 1 2 3	

APPENDIX 5
DIAGNOSTIC ASSESSMENT, CHILD PSYCHIATRY –
MOUNT SINAI MEDICAL CENTER

DATE:_____

CHILD'S NAME: _____ EVALUATOR: _____

1. Diagnosis (DSM III)   a. Major Defense Mechanism:

    Axis I   _____   _____

    Axis II   _____   _____

    Axis III _____   _____

    Axis IV   _____   b. Major Area of Conflict:

    Axis V   _____   _____

                                               _____

2. Psychologicals: _____

    Verbal I.Q._____   a. Diagnosis:_____

    Performance I.Q._____   _____

    Full-Scale I.Q._____   b. Major Dynamics:_____

    Presence of organicity: _____

    Definite-Probable-Possible-None   _____

3. Pediatric Evaluation:

    a. Physical: WNL/Abnormal (specify):_____

    _____

    b. Special Neurological: WNL/Abnormal (specify):_____

    _____

    c. Neurological Consultation: Not Indicated/Indicated (specify):

    _____

    _____

    d. EEG: Not Indicated/Indicated (specify result):_____

    _____

    e. Laboratory Tests: CBC, 12 Channel, VDRL, Tine Test, Urine
        Analysis, Sickle Cell Prep (if WNL, circle test; if test not done,
        mark with an X; if any test is abnormal, specify):_____

    _____

    _____

        Other Laboratory Tests Performed and Results: _____

    _____

    f. Intercurrent Medical Illnesses:_____

    _____

    _____

    g. Other Consultations:_____

    _____

    _____

4. Family Diagnosis (Degree of pathology and organization/disorganization):

_____

_____

_____

5. Speech and Hearing: Not Indicated/Indicated (specify):

   a. Receptive Language_____

   _____

   b. Expressive Language_____

   _____

   c. Speech_____

   _____

   d. Hearing_____

6. Cognitive and Perceptual Battery

   a. Sensory Battery: Not Indicated/Indicated (specify results):

   _____

   _____

   _____

   _____

   _____

   b. Motor: Indicated/Indicated (specify results):

   _____

   _____

   _____

   _____

   _____

   c. Cognitive (Academic Level, Developmental Level, etc.):

   _____

   _____

   _____

   _____

   _____

7. Final Disposition:

   _____

   _____

   _____

   Summary:

   _____

   _____

   _____

   _____

   _____

_____M.D.

APPENDIX 6

CHILD PSYCHIATRY INPATIENT/DAY TREATMENT
MONTH/THREE-MONTH DEVELOPMENTAL OBSERVATIONS
MOUNT SINAI MEDICAL CENTER

CHILD'S NAME:_____ EVALUATORS:_____

DATE:_____ DATE OF LAST EVALUATION:_____

Area	Is Problem Present (circle): 0=No; 1=Possible; 2=Yes; 9=Don't Know	Plan
1. Sensory:		
a. Tactile	0 1 2 9	_____
b. Olfactory and Gustatory	0 1 2 9	_____
c. Vesticular	0 1 2 9	_____
d. Auditory	0 1 2 9	_____
e. Visual	0 1 2 9	_____
2. Gross Motor:	0 1 2 9	_____
3. Fine Motor:	0 1 2 9	_____
4. Speech:	0 1 2 9	_____
5. Language:		
a. Receptive	0 1 2 9	_____
b. Expressive	0 1 2 9	_____
6. Cognitive:		
a. Memory (auditory)	0 1 2 9	_____
b. Memory (visual)	0 1 2 9	_____
c. Left-right orientation	0 1 2 9	_____
d. Attention	0 1 2 9	_____
e. Differentiation, thought from action	0 1 2 9	_____
f. Mode of thinking	0 1 2 9	_____
g. Comprehension, cause and effect	0 1 2 9	_____
7. Specific Learned Skills:		
a. Color	0 1 2 9	_____
b. Time concepts	0 1 2 9	_____
c. Vocabulary	0 1 2 9	_____
d. Writing	0 1 2 9	_____
e. Reading	0 1 2 9	_____
f. Arithmetic	0 1 2 9	_____
g. Money	0 1 2 9	_____
h. General information	0 1 2 9	_____
i. Motivation to learn	0 1 2 9	_____
8. Personal Skills:		
a. Sleeping and wakening	0 1 2 9	_____
b. Toileting	0 1 2 9	_____
c. Eating	0 1 2 9	_____
d. Self-care of everyday needs	0 1 2 9	_____
9. Social:		
a. Level of play	0 1 2 9	_____
b. Relations to children	0 1 2 9	_____
c. Relations to primary therapist	0 1 2 9	_____

	d.	Relations to other staff	0	1	2	9	_____
	e.	Relation to adults in family	0	1	2	9	_____
	f.	Relation to children in family	0	1	2	9	_____
10.	Play and Activity:					
	a.	Appropriateness of/ content of play	0	1	2	9	_____
	b.	Specific likes and dislikes:					

_____   _____

_____

11. Morality:

	a.	Understands good and bad	0	1	2	9	_____
	b.	Acceptance of rules	0	1	2	9	_____
	c.	Has ideals of right and wrong	0	1	2	9	_____

_____

_____ , M.D.

_____

APPENDIX 7

INPATIENT UNIT AND DAY TREATMENT PROGRAM
CHILD PSYCHIATRY DEVELOPMENTAL ASSESSMENT
VIA OBSERVATIONS ON THE MILIEU (Ages are estimates)
MOUNT SINAI MEDICAL CENTER

I. Sensory System

A. Auditory: Does child hear and understand words and language?
    Follow directions? Follows commands? Speech excessively
    loud? Does child over- or underreact to noises or unusual
    sounds? Does child misunderstand or confuse words? (e.g.,
    pen/pin; fish/dish)/ Hallucinations?

B. Visual: Problem with vision; rubs eyes often; blinks often;
    covers one eye when reading or focusing; holds reading closer
    than normal; bumps into objects or people; problem following
    with eyes. Hallucinations? Depth perception: spills glass of
    water; trouble catching ball; confused in open space (e.g.,
    gym).

C. Tactile: Oversensitive to touch. Withdraw from touch? Need
    to touch? Hallucinations?

D. Olfactory and Gustatory: "Funny" smells or tastes?
    Hallucinations?

E. Vesticular: Dizziness? Vestibular stimulation: Rocking?
    Headbanging? Twirling? Posturing? Darting?

II. Action and Ability

A. Manipulation (fine motor and adaptive):
    Stack cubes? Stack toys? Set up dishes?
    Right- or left-handed or ambidextrous?
    Good grasp of pencil when draws or writes (age 4 to 5).
    Uses scissors correctly (age 4 to 5); cuts in straight line?
    Uses knife and fork well (age 5 to 6).
    Goodenough age? Design copy age? 0 + by 3/4.

    ☐ - 4.   △ - 5.   ◇ - 7.

    Reversals of letters — up to age 6 to 7;
    Legibility of handwriting? By 9, joined up and neat.
    By 12, writes well. Sloppy? Trouble positioning paper?
    Can child deal cards: If practice, can do at least by 7/8.
    Catch ball: Arms straight (immature — 4); arms bent at elbows
    (mature). Bounce ball?

B. Locomotion and Gross Motor:

    Any obvious "deformities" (jerky movements of arms and legs,
    toe walking, pigeon walking, other abnormality)?
    Modifies speed well (age 4).
    Tiptoes, hops, use trike (age 4).
    Climbs on monkey bar (age 7).
    By 9 to 10: Can bat ball and catch well.
    Inability to cross midline? (i.e., has to turn body around
                                    completely to catch)
    Most 5-year-olds run 30 yards in < 10 sec; 9 years old in

< 7 sec.
Ball throw: Most 5-year-old boys — 22 feet; 10-year-old boys —
52 feet.

III. Language

A. Receptive:

Follows direction — one command at a time: two, three, or four
(by age 5 should follow complex commands — three or four at
a time, e.g., "Go to the bathroom, brush your teeth, urinate,
wash your hands, and then go to bed." An older child who
doesn't follow complex directions may not be negativistic but
may have a receptive problem and needs one command at a
time, e.g., "Brush your teeth". Later, say: "Urinate", etc.
Prepositions by age 4 (on, under, in front of, behind).

B. Expressive:

Age 4 — four-word sentences; asks questions; tells stories.
Age 5 — five-word sentences; names coins; opposite analogies
(e.g., "if fire is hot, ice is _____.:).   Counts to 20.
Names objects — key, pencil, paper, watch, calendar, ring.
Age 6 — definition of words in terms of use, shape, or general
category: (ball, lake, desk, house, banana, curtain, ceiling).

IV. Speech

Age 4 — 90% intelligible. Age 5 — 100% intelligible.
Slurring? Lisping? Stuttering? Infantile pattern (baby talk)?
Mutism? Elective? Rapid or slow speech? Loud? Hoarse?

V. Cognitive

(How the child uses ideas, symbols, and thoughts; integrates
experiences; manipulates objects; and acts in accordance with
knowledge.)

A. Time and Space:

Age 4 — tomorrow/yesterday, am/pm. Age 5 — days of the
week. Age 7 — what time it is; calendar organization; seasons.
Age 8 — months of the year; what year it is; irreversibility of
death; can understand that something that goes faster will take
less time than something that goes slower.

Age 4 — colors. By age 7, learned R.L on self and by age 8,
R.L on others.
By age 5 differentiates between thought and action. This
process begins at about age 2 and depends on the development
of language and interaction with people in the environment.
May still consider dreams, thoughts, and fantasies as tangible
reality, e.g., parent says, "Did you take the cookie?" Child
says "No." This was neither "stealing" nor "lying." The
child had the wish for the cookie, therefore took it. When
caught he wished he hadn't taken it because parent is angry,
therefore said no, i.e., wish = reality (see Morality — age 5).

The child learns that his thoughts do not influence environment,
e.g., "angry thought did not cause person to be hurt."

By this age (5) the child recognizes need for causal sources even if not correct, e.g., "smoke makes the engine go"; "How does the bicycle go?: — With wheels". Later on (7/8), "The bike goes with wheels and the boy makes them work by pedaling", i.e., more accurate knowledge of causes.

B. Sorting and Relating Objects:

Age 4/5 — begin to sort objects in groups and apply language, e.g., pants and shirts are clothes.

Age 7/8 — more complicated classes, e.g., objects that float and sink, hard substances vs. soft substances, various tastes.

Age 9/10 — multiple classes and relationships, e.g., plastic utensils as compared to metal utensils, types of large vehicles vs. small ones, classify types of animals — domesticated, pets, wild, etc.

C. Conservation:

Age 8 — quantity: if same amount of milk is in a tall, skinny glass vs. a small, fat glass, child knows it's the same.

Age 9/10 weight: a pound is a pound — younger child couldn't understand that a pound of feathers (light) = a pound of cement (heavy).

Age 11/12 — volume.

D. Reversibility:

Age 7/8 $3 + 2 = 5$, therefore $5 - 2 = 3$ or $5 - 3 = 2$.
When child plays games he can therefore begin to backtrack what happened. Casino is a game that requires manipulation of numbers back and forth.

Age 12 — thinking about problems is the important developmental factor, e.g., tries to figure out why a plant died.
Games such as backgammon requires thinking out the moves. Still concrete.

Age 13 — more symbolic thoughts — proportions, ratios, percentages, probabilities.
Reading level? Math level? Comprehension? Judgment?

VI. Personal

Age 4 — Dress and undress (except buttons, back fastenings, laces); own toilet needs.

Age 5 — Almost complete independence in everyday acts; simple errands; helps in house.

Age 6 — Manages own daily care.
    7 — May get self to school.
    9 — Reliability in helping tasks.
    12 — Rebelliousness, critical parents.

VII. Social Form of Play

Age 3 or younger, solitary play; age 4, parallel play; 5, project play (all do same activity); 6/7, "cooperative" play; 9 and on (peak 12), "competitive" play.
Age 4 — tolerance of short separation and waiting.

Age 5 – more confident about himself; picks friends and peers.
Age 6 – understands needs of others.
Age 7 – greater link to peer group.
Age 8 – needs acceptance by peers; resents isolation.
Age 9 – single sex groups.

VIII. Play/Activity

Age 3 or less – dolls, water, sand.
Age 4 – imaginative, takes adult role, "oedipal" play.
Age 5 – "king of castle," dress-up, make-believe, tall tales,
building and destruction, deals with fears and phobias in play.
Age 6 – games, tag, puppets.
Age 7 – begins collecting, hobbies, ring-a-lievo.
Age 8 – family romance and twin fantasies, loves fairy tales –
        identifies with the "good" characters – wants the bad
        ones punished.
Age 9 – decreased interest in fairy tales, tag games become
        more complicated.
Age 9 on + – increased awareness of upcoming puberty, especially
        in girls.
Age 12 – team games.

IX. Morality

Age 4 – understands good and bad; bouts of quarrelsomeness.
Age 5 – begins to accept rules – before this occurs one cannot
        play a game (checkers, cards) with the child and make
        him play by the rules. Until the idea of rules are
        established, the child is dominated by the idea that he
        has to win all the time (see Cognitive: Differentiate
        thought/fantasy).
Age 6 – rules become more important.
Age 6 to 7 – "harsh" superego, i.e., very strict about what is
        right and wrong (Piaget: "moral realism"). Child will
        want another child who was bad to be punished severely,
        i.e., identification with the aggressor. Have to be
        careful not to play into this tendency many children have.
        Child "projects his guilt," i.e., "he did it," or "you did
        it" when accused of wrongdoing.
Age 7 to 8 – ideals of right and wrong. Parents and teachers are
        still "all powerful." Is child unable to accept rules?
Age 8 on – "less harsh" superego. Idea of justice and cooperation.
        Child can understand that infraction was accidental, for
        example, or that child was much younger or sicker or
        retarded and therefore shouldn't apply strict punishment
        for wrongdoing. Is there a failure to develop sense of
        right/wrong? Does child consciously steal or lie?
Age 12 – rebellion.

X. Familial Support (or undermining of age-appropriate tasks)

e.g., mother who doesn't allow child to separate or function
        independently
e.g., father who forces his 7-year-old child to learn how to bat
        even though he doesn't have the skills yet
e.g., parent of retarded child who encourages the child to do to
        his capacity but not beyond

XI.   Child's Emotional Reactions, Thinking and other symptoms which interfere with age-appropriate skills

  e.g., 8-year-old aggressive child who can't be in peer group
  e.g., 9-year-old distractible child who hasn't learned how to write well
  e.g., depressed child who can't participate in tasks
  e.g., negativistic child who refuses to cooperate

XII. Estimate of Whether Fixation or Regression (and whether able to progress to age appropriate level)

  e.g., 7-year-old whose mother died and regresses to solitary play
  e.g., 12-year-old retarded child whose maximum goal would be a 6 year level across the board
  e.g., child with environmental deprivation who can increase skills almost to age-appropriate levels

INDEX